Homo Sapiens

Volume III: Confrontations of Cultures

A Collection of Essays on Superstition, Faith, Religion and Politics

Shimon Garber

Contents

Shimon Garber © 2021
Newcomers Authors Publishing Group
All rights reserved

Second edition

Russian Text Editor: Anna Pelan
Corrector: V. Belinker
Designer: Paul Hawkins

TX 8-821-907
ISBN: 978-1-950430-369 (Hard cover)
ISBN: 978-1-950430-376 (eBook)

Unless specified, all Scripture is taken from the New King James Version®. Copyright © 1982 by Thomas Nelson. It has been used with permission.

The books of the *Homo Sapiens* series:
ISBN: 978-1-950430345; HS I&II; HC; Eng
ISBN: 978-1-950430-352; HS I&II; EPUB; Eng
ISBN: 978-1-950430-369; HS III; HC; Eng
ISBN: 978-1-950430-376; HS III; EPUB; Eng

Dear reader—

This book is a translation from an original manuscript written in Russian, and like any translation, it only partially captures the spirit of the original. However, it might still offer a glimpse into what life was like for an immigrant during the last decades of the twentieth century.

All written essays express the author's personal opinion on all topics.

The author

PREFACE

Dear Reader:

The collection of various essays written at different times and on seemingly different topics combines a single theme: the species of *Homo sapiens,* its development, history, and a unique experiment of biological nature, which created a fantastic phenomenon—the human race.

In some chapters, we must return to the distant past of our species' origin and the emergence of different civilizations. It is done for the narrative's logical construction to avoid the impression of separately torn pieces unrelated to each other and to make it more interesting for readers.

The third book of *Homo Sapiens* is a logical continuation of our species' history in the modern world. The world is divided by countries, religions, and ideologies. Despite the declared principles of universal equality and the obligation to defend peace and prosperity, there is still the danger of a military solution to confrontations. Modern weapons and technology could destroy peoples and even entire countries with appalling cruelty. The history of slavery runs through all stages of the development of our species. In some countries, slavery still exists.

The future of our species depends on how we deal with it today. We are living on the same planet. Will our species find a path of reconciliation and forgiveness now?

The biological nature of man is manifested in his behavioral motives. However, man is a social being. He cannot live outside of society. A person is born with an already-formed brain, having certain instincts embedded in the brain's limbic system. A person acquires social skills in the development process, communicating with the surrounding society.

Due to climate change, relatively recently, by historical standards, about sixty to ninety thousand years ago, some scientists count as three hundred thousand years ago, the human species came out of Africa, together with other groups of animals, in search of favorable habitats. Scientists tell us there were at least twenty different types of people, but our species, *Homo sapiens*, survived.

Despite the large brain, our species, *Homo sapiens*, followed not the heart's command but a primitive biological instinct. The brain needs to be fed. The brain does not care how and from where the food might come. It could come from other animals or a neighbor. The brain has no ethics. It merely performs the biological function of survival. The blood flow through the brain should bring lipids, proteins, and sugar. The brain takes what it needs; the rest and metabolic waste are carried away.

Our specie created civilizations five millennia ago and has gone incredibly far from primitive hunter-gatherers to the conquerors of space in a relatively short period. Millennia passed, and the species of Homo sapiens settled worldwide and began to move to a sedentary lifestyle. In this evolutionary process, our brains lost 50 to 250 cubic centimeters, but we learned to study and understand the processes in our brains.

We owe survival on this planet to our brain and our ability to understand the processes that allow our consciousness to remain human without returning to our wild past condition. But what happened during WWI and WWII created awareness of the similarity to wild animal behavior.

In the past, we have experienced terrible cataclysms, extermination wars, and disappearances of nations, civilizations, and races. We passed through terrifying epidemics that took millions of lives. Cruel religious strifes led to wars on a planetary scale. Civil wars brought devastation, poverty, and massive loss of innocent people—world wars had monstrous numbers of victims. Five millennia seems an unimaginably colossal time, but historically it is negligible for the *Homo sapiens* species' evolutionary changes.

The transition from a communal-clan community of gatherers and hunters, living a nomadic way of life, to sedating and creating the first permanent settlements, later called the emergence of the first civilizations, was a gigantic step. The availability of fresh water, material for the construction of dwellings, and fertile soil for the cultivation of crops are necessary conditions for the emergence of such civilizations.

Creating iconic public worship houses allowed priests of various early forms of religion to create communities worshipping the new common deity.

People came here for public ceremonial prayers and sacrificial ceremonies. People created jewelry, sculptures, and images of worshipped gods.

The cults of specific deities often became the center of social life. There was a stratification of society along with property and social grounds.

The land and the canals supplying fresh water were declared the property of the deity of the given settlement, and the priests became servants, fulfilling the will of the deities.

There was a tax burden for the use of land and water. Violation of obligations was often punishable by transfer to debt captivity. A person could be ordered to work for a certain period for the debt, or it was possible to pay it off by giving one's child into slavery.

The tradition of appointing (crowning) temporary warlords survived into the future in subsequent religions. Priests might appoint warlords to attack or defend against nomads during the war. Prisoners captured during wars were turned into enslaved people.

Homo sapiens migrated and expanded about sixty to ninety thousand years ago (but more and more new findings of the dates are coming up, such last finding in Morocco, dated 300 000 years ago) until they inhabited almost the entire planet. Our species, at the age of reproductive maturation (girls at around thirteen years, boys at around fourteen years), strive to continue reproducing the species. In addition to instinctive physiological needs, many people tend to dominate and stand out from their environment. Domination is linked to the law of nature inherited from our ancestors, apes. The need for superiority over other individuals is an instinctive desire to take a leading place in society, allowing have more food and higher status to feel superior to others.

Centuries and millennia have passed, and many civilizations have appeared and disappeared. Cities and fortresses were built. All new waves of conquerors came and destroyed what was created by the previous civilization. Newcomers built their temples. The species of *Homo sapiens* created art and architectural wonders, discovered unexplored secrets of sciences and created the latest weapons capable of destroying all living things. Humans stepped on the moon. In the twenty-first century, the world's population surpassed eight billion people.

Our society is built on biological principles. Just as they did millennia ago, our species worship their gods and prepare to destroy those who pray to other gods. Dominant people lead our populations, backed by religious leaders. Leaders are appointed by God (all power from God) or elected democratically; religion or ideology confirms the government's existing system's legitimacy. Religions and ideologies change, but the essence remains.

Our society is divided into dominants, adaptives, and outlaws.

THE HISTORY OF
SLAVERY

We can consider slavery part of the long history of the species of *Homo sapiens*. Climate change in Africa has forced much wildlife, including hominids, to search for favorable alternative habitats. Our species' exodus from Africa is probably since the beginning of this species, judging by the remains of early representatives of *Homo sapiens* found in Israel.

The large brain allowed numerous populations of *Homo sapiens* to explore vast expanses of the planet. They fought predators, other hominid species, wildlife, natural disasters, diseases, and hunger. They survived thanks to the ability to share food. The maternal instinct to feed one's young exists in all types of surviving animals. However, sharing food with members of the population, even the old ones, which does not obviously benefit society, as a whole, allowed our species to become humans.

Homo sapiens left the African cradle. The search for food and more favorable conditions for living forced them to act.

Extreme conditions in the wild, with dangerous, multiple hungry enemies, have occurred for thousands of years. The brain, which reached a volume of 1,650 cubic centimeters, the only natural weapon of our distant ancestors, has adapted and developed, saving the specie from destruction. The ability to use fire, create tools, fight predators and other hominids' representatives honed the ability to survive. These were populations of hunter-gatherers subject to totem rites and taboos. Dominating all the new spaces, the populations of *Homo sapiens* moved further and further, spreading across the planet. They settled almost all continents and most large islands for several thousand years.

The population of hunter-gatherers' transition to a sedentary lifestyle is associated with understanding the benefits of growing crops on the coasts of full-flowing rivers. Instead of long and complex searches for food, there was an opportunity to grow crops and make stocks for adverse weather conditions.

Settling in one place changed the whole way of tribal life. Settlements with temples were built to worship the deities of the tribe. The dominant leader became the priest of a temple dedicated to a particular deity. Values appeared: land, water, housing, grain supplies, livestock, and enslaved people. Domesticated livestock and grain reserves made it possible to increase the family without fear of hunger.

Slavery has existed almost continually in the history of *Homo sapiens.* Even in the community tribal society, enslaved people were subordinate to the dominant leader and his assistant shamans' will.

In the transition to a sedentary way of life and temples' construction, slavery was a logical phenomenon, and enslaved people might come from both those in debt and prisoners captured in various wars. Enslaved people became valuable because they were used in different jobs. They dug irrigation canals, built ziggurat temples, and did other work.

In all likelihood, the world owes the appearance of writing to temples. Cuneiform writing appeared due to this need. It was used for recording taxes, accounting for stocks, and calculating the number of enslaved people required to create a system capable of storing it.

Our species' brain volume loss may have existed since the formation of settlements that prescribe behavior, worship, and submission rules. The worship of various pagan gods replaced the rules of taboos and totems. Suppression, obedience, and the proclaimed rules deprived the members of the community initiative and desired to resist. Fear of death or punishment as expulsion from the settlement suppressed the initiative. To be expelled from the community meant death or capture by strangers. The adaptable and helpful ones survived.

CIVILIZATION

About six thousand years ago, in Mesopotamia, cities began to emerge along the Tigris and Euphrates rivers, erected by people who arrived on ships, calling themselves "black-headed." We know them as Sumerians. They could be coming from India.

The place from the valleys of the Indus River, India, has given the world a wealth of knowledge and new nationalities. It could be the cradle of civilized communities that came many groups of people with knowledge, which allowed the existing population to make significant progress in various areas. From India came the Gypsies and Aryan tribes (Indo-Iranians). In addition to much other knowledge, the Sumerians built ziggurats—temples for their many pagan gods. The demonic Adolf Hitler considered the ancient Aryans the German nation's ancestors.

In Mesopotamia, priests who served in Sumerian temples were part of the dominant class, which owned allotments. They controlled irrigation canals, chose warlords in case of war, collected taxes, and rented out small land plots.

On larger farms, enslaved people received little food for their work. Tenants gave most of the harvest to the temples, living on the rest. For non-payment of rent or taxes, tenants became debt-enslaved people. They could pay by giving their child away as payment for a debt.

It was one of the first societies to use enslaved labor. Hunter-gatherers had no enslaved people; they did not lead a sedentary lifestyle, moving in search of the necessary food. The transition to a sedentary way of life and the creation of the first city-states led to slavery, social stratification, and the emergence of a caste of priests serving the cult of the gods.

Slavery accompanied the entire history of the civilization of the human community.

Captives captured during wars, debtors who could not return borrowed money, and criminals caught red-handed were enslaved. In a primitive communal existence, women were taken into slavery, and men were killed or sacrificed to the totem, then eaten during the meal.

Slavery developed during the construction of cities with a central temple to worship deities. Slavery was used in societies dependent on agricultural production.

Here the work of enslaved people was economically justified. Forced labor was used to construct temples, fortresses, protective walls, and canals. Enslaved people were used in domestic, agricultural, or building work.

The Semitic Akkadian tribes conquered Schumer's cities. Legend says that Sargon (real name unknown) was a gardener for one of the kings but killed the king and took his place. Sargon's name (meaning *'legitimate'*) came to us with a clay plaque where he called himself "King of Schumer and Akkad."

Babylon was subordinated to the Semitic tribal union of Chaldea. The rulers of Assyria and Babylon subsequently used this title. The Semitic nomads, the Akkads who conquered Sumeria, took over the cities.

Akkad's tribes conquered Sumer's city-states and accepted their culture, polytheism, and praying at ziggurats. The Sumerians were assimilated, and the Akkadian language was widely adopted.

Ziggurats had no interior, and prayers were held on the upper level. There was a different elevation on the upper square of the temple—the place of the deity. Similar dwellings for the gods were built in other religions. The engravings of the Temple of Solomon in the Jewish religion bear a resemblance to the Sumerian ziggurats. Such a holy place, a separate room for God to stay, was allowed to be entered only by the high priest once a year. Like ziggurats, prayer temples were

built in Central America, where human sacrifices were
made at the top of such ziggurats. The Mausoleum of
the leader of the world proletariat, Vladimir Lenin,
was built in the form of a ziggurat; inside is a coffin
with a glass lid, revealing the mummified body of the
leader. He is still admired by many, waiting in a long
queue to see the appearance of the man who died in
1924.

Simultaneously, the Mesopotamian Crescent
existed Hittites, Phoenicians, Philistines, Amores,
Ivusei, and many others. Fertile land helped developed
city-states in the Middle East along the Mediterranean
Sea coast. These city-states were engaged in maritime
trade, agriculture, and crafts. The Torah mentions
bloody wars between the Semites and the Philistines.
The Semitic tribes of nomadic herders, who invaded
Canaan, waged long-term wars over the territories.
They worshipped various gods, Baal, Asherah, and
Astare.

Judaism, as a monotheistic religion, competed with
many other cults. After the fall of Judea, made by the
Babylonian king Nebuchadnezzar II began Babylonian
captivity, where some small group of religious leaders
developed the concept of a single God, Yahweh.
Yahweh became a single God of the Kindom of Judea.

Torah prescribed a gentle and fair attitude towards
enslaved people. Slavery as a way of creating values is

mentioned in the founding Torah, which entered the Old Testament of the Judeo-Christian religion.

Although the enslaved people were the property of the master, the Torah forbade maiming the enslaved person. Enslaved people included children sold into slavery by their parents for debts, prisoners of war, or people bought from other nations. For example, the Phoenicians traded enslaved people.

The murder of an enslaved person was punishable. It was forbidden to maim enslaved; if this law was violated, the enslaved person should be given freedom. Enslaved women were often concubines; it was forbidden to sell them, and they were supposed to be released freely. Enslaved people were supposed to be released after six years. Still, if an enslaved person married during a slavery period, had a family, and did not want to leave his wife and children, that meant the enslaved person refused freedom.

In the third millennium BC, in Egypt, the Ancient and Middle Kingdoms built tombs—pyramids for pharaohs. Egyptian priests created monumental pyramids for their pharaohs. They were considered the deities' earthly governors, and the mummified corpses were buried inside the pyramids with incredible pomp. The labor of forced enslaved people was widely used during the construction of the pyramids.

Religious leaders believed in an afterlife because it allowed them to convince their flock of the need for goodness and worship of the designated deity, securing a place in the afterlife. To serve in the other world of the deceased rulers, those left behind were supposed to prepare everything needed in the mortal world, including enslaved people. The disobedient and blasphemers were threatened with eternal torment and suffering in the concentration camp of otherworldly life.

Babylon in the nineteenth century BC was subordinated to the tribes of the Amorites. The main cult temple, the Tower of Babel, was dedicated to the god Marduk.

The most famous ruler is Hammurabi, known for his laws carved on the basalt obelisk (now kept in the Louvre). Some of these laws became the Ten Commandments in the Torah.

Power passed to the Assyrian Dynasty. Assyria conquered Babylon and continued in conquest wars, increasing income and many new enslaved people for constructing walls and temples-ziggurats to honor the designated deities. Under attack from various tribes, New Babylon's rulers allied with the northern Assyrian neighbors.

In 732—722 BC, Assyrian king Sargon II waged war with the northern kingdom of Israel. He captured and took into slavery the *"ten tribes"* of northern Israel. In place of the hijacked inhabitants in Judea-Samaria, the region was resettled by people from other conquered territories.

Ten tribes of Jews from Israel were scattered

among other nations and lost forever. Modern Israel continues to search for its once-lost brothers, occasionally calling certain peoples the lost tribes of the Jews and even resettling some of them to modern Israel.

The southern kingdom of Judah also did not escape captivity. Assyrian king Nebuchadnezzar II, the second king of the Neo-Babylon, invaded Judea's southern kingdom in 598 B.C. and took the Jews captive. The population of conquered Judea was sent to Babylon. The temple in Jerusalem was destroyed. In 539 B.C., the Persian king Cyrus the Great conquered Babylonia and allowed numerous captive peoples to return to their homelands.

Africa's Black population has always been attractive prey for slave traders. Arab slave people traders took them from Africa to Arabia, the Ottoman Empire, Persia, and Egypt. Captured enslaved people were transported to Egypt, Phoenicia, Greece, and Rome.

Armed squads of slave traders hunted Black African populations across the continent. The enslaved-people trade was essential to the economies of such states as the Arab Caliphate, the Golden Horde, the Crimean Khanate, and the Ottoman Empire.

The slave-owning system existed in the history of many states. An enslaved person could become free under certain circumstances. The Old Testament describes the rules for treating enslaved people by liberation from slavery after a certain period. Slavery existed in ancient Rome, where the gladiator, a survivor of many battles in the circus arena, could be awarded the gift of freedom from Caesar.

The institution of freedmen existed in many countries. Although they became citizens, enslaved people who were ransomed or freed were obliged to comply with many conditions limiting their rights.

Enslaved people sometimes rose against their enslavers, hoping to gain freedom. Such uprisings were suppressed with particular cruelty. Slavery existed throughout almost the entire history of humankind. Enslaved people's labor was used in ancient Egypt's agricultural work and construction of pyramids. Ancient Rome, Greece, and Mesopotamian states owned enslaved people. Enslaved people's labor was used in domestic work. There were also privileged classes of enslaved people whose knowledge or talents could be useful for the owners' benefit.

Islam—Slavery—
Religious Wars

In the early seventh century, a man appeared in the Arabian Peninsula in the Arab city of Medina. He founded a new religion called Islam. It was an Abrahamic religion, just like Judaism and Christianity. The new prophet, Muhammad, did recognize prophets Ibrahim (Abraham), Musa (Moses), Isa (Jesus), Jebrail (Gabriel), and others. Muhammad believed his family was Ishmael's descendants, Abraham's son and servant Hagar. The people of Medina did not accept him, and Muhammad was forced to move to Mecca. There was a large black obelisk, which has been considered sacred since ancient times. The city became sacred for Islam's followers, and the tradition of pilgrimage to the city and worship of the sacred stone is still preserved.

Islam was able to unite the many disparate tribes of Arabs living in the Arabian Peninsula as unified followers of the prophet Muhammad and create a powerful army that sought to conquer and establish an Arab Caliphate. Slavery in Islam has its roots in the pre-Islamic era.

Islam allows slavery, considering the release of an enslaved person a godly deed. A harem with slave concubines is allowed in Islam. Even during Muhammad's life, the victorious offensive of Muslim Arabs began. Having conquered Arabia, the Arabs captured territories in Asia, north and north-west Africa, the Near East, Egypt, Persia, the Caucasus, Central Asia, the Mediterranean islands, southern Italy, and the Iberian Peninsula.

The Ottoman Empire formed a Muslim state in Anatolia in the thirteenth century. By the beginning of the eighth century, the Arab Caliphate had been completed. Millions of prisoners were sold into slavery. In the Muslim world, the conquest of vast territories and states created the traditions of the slave trade of captured masses of people. Wikipedia cites rough figures of enslaved people in Muslim territories as between 11.5 and 14 million people (conquered vast territories 632 —1517). Slave labor was used in mining, irrigation, cattle breeding, and households. The Arab slave trade flourished in west Asia and north and southeast Africa. Slavery exists in Islamic countries: Chad, Mauritania, Mali, and Sudan. Until the beginning of the eighth century, the Crimean Khanate was engaged in a mass slave trade (the central market of the slave trade, the city of Kafa, (today Theodosia) with the Ottoman Empire.

Ukrainian hetmans, Circassians, Novgorod planters, Cossacks of Peter the Great, Vikings, Byzantines, Italian, Genoese, and Venetian merchants carried out the enslaved-people trade. The main buyers were Muslims from Egypt, Syria, Anatolia, and Persia.

In the Ottoman Empire, slavery was legal, and in the slave markets of Constantinople (Istanbul), a fifth of the population was enslaved. The Arab or Islamic enslaved-people trade began in the middle of the seventh century and lasted fourteen centuries. Sexual slavery in the Ottoman Empire continued until the early twentieth century.

Since the purchase and sale of Muslims were prohibited under Islam's law, the primary "goods" were enslaved people from Africa, residents of the Asian steppes, the North Caucasus population, Lithuania's principality, the Polish kingdom, and Russia.

The invasions of the Tatar-Mongols hordes marked the beginning of the thirteenth century under Genghis Khan's leadership.

Central Asia was conquered from the Indus to the Caspian Sea. The ruin of cities and settlements accompanied captivity and slavery during the Tatar-Mongolian conquest. The inhabitants of the cities taken by storm left after a terrible massacre was driven out into the field and divided among the soldiers who turned them into slavery. The prisoners were used in the siege of cities. During the city's siege, prisoners filled the ditches at the city walls. The prisoners who survived the massacre were sold into slavery. Women were raped, and wealthy townspeople were tortured, extorting money. Women, children, and artisans were taken as prisoners. A significant number of the captives were sold in the large enslaved-people markets. There are numerous literary sources by Arab, Persian, Turkish, and Armenian authors from the thirteenth to the fifteenth centuries.

The role of most significant international enslaved —people market was Crimea, including the city of Sudak, Constantinople in Europe, and Alexandria in North Africa.

The enslaved-people trade in Western Europe also existed in the Middle Ages, run by Scandinavian Vikings and Italian merchants from Genoa and Venice. Also, enslaved people were imported by the Portuguese. In the eleventh century, the Irish city of Dublin was Western Europe's largest enslaved people market. The gradual transition from slavery to serfdom lasted for several centuries. Slavery was permitted by law, but the Christian Church actively opposed the enslavement of fellow Christians. Muslim Spain Al-Andalus imported many enslaved people and was a transit point for sending enslaved people to Muslim countries.

Slavery was an essential part of the Ottoman

Empire. The Ottoman Wars in Europe brought a large number of enslaved Christians. Captive enslaved people converted to Islam and were trained to serve in the sultan's army. Usually of Christian origin, women were selected as Sultan's concubines. A famous example was Roxolana, the beloved wife of Suleiman the Magnificent.

In Kievan Rus and Russia itself, enslaved people were classified as servants. The Tsarist Decree of 1581 prohibited the removal of peasants from a landowner without his permission. Peasants living there were assigned to the landowner along with the land. By decree of Peter the Great in 1723, the domestic enslaved people were transferred to serfs.

Slavery existed throughout the Kingdom of Poland. There were enslaved people who could be punished and sold. In Scandinavia, slavery was abolished in the nineteenth century.

British Wales, Ireland, and Scotland were the last areas of Christian Europe to abolish the institutions of slavery. The enslaved people trade in England was officially abolished in 1102. Everywhere slavery passed into feudal serfdom. In both cases, the peasants have forced laborers and worked hard to benefit their masters. They were excluded from the judicial system and were the property of their masters. Enslaved people had no personal property. The serfs were given plots of land on which they were obliged to work, were paid a certain amount, and had the opportunity to accumulate for themselves some surpluses. Such privileges did not exist for enslaved people. Serfs could have a family, but the owners could sell family members to another owner. Serfdom gradually fell into decay. The economy of commodity-money relations and the inflation that took place pushed for monetary payments instead of subsistence farming.

Lack of food, weakened immunity, numerous epidemics, military disasters, and civil wars have caused poverty, vagrancy, unsanitary conditions, and the spread of lice, fleas, and rats.

The abolition of serfdom occurred in different countries, depending on the economic situation. A plague epidemic broke out in Europe in the middle of the fourteenth century, claiming nearly half of the population. The climate of Europe had changed significantly to colder and more humid.

Devastated landowners could sell the land to serfs and liberation from serfdom.

Epidemics have occurred in many countries in both the West and East. The plague escalated into a pandemic, penetrating along with ships filled with enslaved people. Throughout Europe, frantic crowds were looking for the culprits of the pandemic. Jews had become victims of widespread hysteria. Mass pogroms, murders, burning at the stake, and the mockery of corpses were an everyday occurrence. Jews were hanged and burned, hunted with dogs, and drowned in rivers.

There was no consensus on the cause of the infection. It was called an unknown virus, anthrax bacillus, Mongolian plague, and pneumonic diseases.

Epidemics led to a significant reduction in the population. Such a situation brought changes in feudal relations. Small artisans began to hire people. Fields, which were sown with crops, turned into pastures for livestock.

Taxes increased, and the boundaries between estates were blurred. In Europe, riots and uprisings brutally suppressed led to the transition from feudal to rental relations in agriculture. Replacing serfdom with a quitrent (meaning a substantial portion of whatever was made) became a more progressive economic system.

COLONIALISM

The crusade proclaimed in France by Pope Urban II in 1096 took a series of military campaigns to take Jerusalem and the Holy Land back from Muslim control. After many attempts at conquering Jerusalem, many territories of the Middle East, the countries on the Syrian coast of the Mediterranean Sea, and North African countries, France's colonial policy began. Vast territories became French colonies.

Great geographical discoveries in the fifteenth and sixteenth centuries connected European countries' desire to find new trade routes with India. From there, the spices were commonly believed to have come to Europe. The Arabs monopolized this trade and did not admit strangers to it. The fifteenth century began with the process of the emergence of capitalist relations.

The peasants were transformed into wage workers

and the means of production, and monetary wealth into capital. According to Karl Marx, the era of primitive accumulation became the threshold of capitalist socio-economic formation.

The Renaissance and great geographical discoveries were approaching at the end of the fifteenth century. The growth of commodity production and the lack of precious metals made Europeans equip sea expeditions to search for new lands.

1488, Portuguese explorers Diego Kahn, Bartolomeu Dias, and others explored Africa's western and southern coasts.

1492—1494, Christopher Columbus discovered America, the Bahamas, and the Antilles.

1497—1499, Vasco da Gama opened a sea route from Western Europe around South Africa to India.

1498—1502 Christopher Columbus, Monso de Ojeda, and Amerigo Vespucci explored the northern coast of South America, its eastern (Brazilian) coast, and the Caribbean coast of Central America.

1513—1525, the Spaniards crossed the Isthmus of Panama, reached the Pacific Ocean, discovered the Gulf of La Plata, the Florida Peninsula, and the Yucatan Peninsula, explored the Gulf Coast, and conquered Mexico and explored the Atlantic coast of South America.

1519—1522, Ferdinand Magellan made the world's first circumnavigation.

1526—1552, Spaniards Francisco Pizarro, Diego

de Almagro, Pedro de Valdivia, G. Quesada, and Francisco de Orellana discovered the Pacific coast of South America. Spain and Portugal claimed a monopoly in acquiring new, previously unknown lands.

The pope's bull in 1454 gave Portugal all rights to the land discovered on the African continent. After the first of Columbus's voyages, the king of Spain asked for the pope's throne to secure all the lands discovered.

Portuguese explorer Enrique "The Navigator" studied the coast of West Africa during sea expeditions. As a result of numerous expeditions, the Portuguese established control of the African coast. Portugal, in 1420, captured the island of Madeira and then the Azores. In 1520, the Portuguese discovered Brazil. By the sixteenth century, Portugal owned numerous colonial territories in India, spice islands in Southeast Asia, more land in the Persian Gulf, and territory in West Africa.

Portugal established control on the coasts of continents and islands, where fortresses and factories were built. Exploiting captured colonies brought considerable profits to the treasury of the monarchy. The Portuguese actively enslaved people, buying them from local African princes or capturing them by force. Enslaved people were sold and used in the New World and on islands, growing coffee, cocoa, sugar, and tobacco. The Portuguese exported gold, silver, and ivory. They controlled most of the Atlantic enslaved people's markets. The most famous Portuguese conquistadors (conquerors) were Aretha de Albuquerque and Filipe de Brito e Nicote.

In 1492, Christopher Columbus discovered America. In the middle of the sixteenth century, Spain dominated the American continent. Vast streams of silver and gold poured into the Spanish royal treasury from the conquered American colonies.

Spanish caravels were carrying full holds of new goods previously unknown in Europe. Pirates chased the caravels, and Spain created a colossal fleet to protect the sailors, calling it the Great or Invincible Armada.

Spanish colonial possessions were distributed in North, Central, and South America, Africa, the Caribbean islands, Florida, and Jamaica.

Conquistadors of Spain were the youngest children in the family. Under the inheritance law, all property was passed to the eldest heir. All other sons received swords and blessings to win their place under the sun.

Hernan Cortez landed with six hundred people in what is now Mexico. It was a powerful Aztec empire with a multimillion population.

Francisco Pizarro captured the Inca Empire in Peru. Pedro de Alvarado and Lieutenant Cortez destroyed the Mayan Empire.

Diego de Almagro, the partner of Francisco Pizarro, opened modern Chile.

One of three brothers, Gonzalo Pizarro, rebelled against Spanish rule and was executed.

The treasury of the Spanish kings received gems, gold, silver, spices, and pearls. Spanish caravels crossed the ocean into Guadalquivir's river with full-flowing water and climbed up to Seville.

The valuables they brought were handed over to customs. Many lists of that have survived even today.

The British Empire became the world's most immense colonial power, displacing territories on all five continents. The British colonialists took part in the business of the Portuguese. They bought gold, silver, and ivory from the Portuguese. British corporations, as well as French ones, drove the Portuguese out of the African colonies. England created a powerful fleet and became the Lady of the Seas, competing with Spain, which created the great Armada to protect its caravels, carrying gold, silver, tea, tobacco, and raw materials to produce various goods.

England extended its rule to the northern American states, Canada, Australia, New Zealand, India, Singapore, China, Ireland, and many others.

Colonial possessions were suppliers of raw materials for the metropolis. The British cities of Bristol and Liverpool became the largest suppliers of enslaved people from Africa to America.

England and Holland allied to oust Portugal from the spice trade. England secured India, and Holland had the advantage in the spice trade from the Indonesian archipelago.

France, like most European countries, was involved

in colonial conquests. The French colonies' empire began in July 1605 in North America (now Nova Scotia, Canada.) France colonized many territories in northern Africa. They won territories in West and equatorial Africa, Madagascar, New Caledonia, Guadeloupe, Martinique, Guiana, Senegal, and India.

France owned vast territories in Canada. The French founded a large colony in North America, New France, Florida, and Louisiana—also several islands in the Caribbean, including French Guyana.

Dutch Colonial Empire: The following list of colonial territories managed by the West-Indies and East-India companies and the North Company does not include the territories annexed by Holland in the nineteenth and twentieth centuries. It competed with the British Empire. It lost to England territories in North America, including New York.

In West Africa, some states.

In North America, New Amsterdam (New York). Several islands in the Caribbean. Many islands in South America.

In South Asia, territories and islands. Some of the territories in the Far East.

In South Africa, the island of Mauritius and vast areas.

The German Colonial Empire was formed in early 1880. The German Colonial Union concluded a treaty with Samoa in 1879. It captured Cameroon, a massive part of Southwest Africa's coast, part of New Guinea, the northern part of the Solomon Islands, and the territory on the coast of East Africa: Marshall Islands, Togo, an area in Kenya, Congo: Territories in Africa, Oceania, and China. After the defeat in the First World War, all colonial possessions were transferred under The Treaty of Versailles to the victorious countries.

The Belgian Colonial Empire was created in 1870, separating from the Netherlands in 1830. Territories: Congo (Zaire), Rwanda-Urundi in East Africa, territories in Central Africa, concession in China's Tianjin, Guatemala in America, attempts to gain a foothold on the coast of Brazil, a colony in Argentina (Entre Rios province)—attempts to gain a foothold in Crete, Borneo, Philippines, New Guinea, and Fiji.

Sweden owned a colony in North America on the banks of the Delaware River.

Russia did not avoid conquering the American colonies, Alaska and Fort Ross. Russia sold Alaska to the US government for $7.2 million in gold in 1867.

Fort Ross in California has been offered for sale many times due to unprofitability. The California earthquake in 1906 destroyed everything except the house of the last commandant. Fort Ross passed from hand to hand.

The discovery of the Americas led to the heyday of the enslaved-people trade of black people from Africa. The enslaved-people trade's central markets were Morocco, Algeria, Tripoli, Cairo, Genoa, and Venice.

The seaside town of Lagos, Portugal, where enslaved Africans were sold, was opened in 1444.

Most countries signed the UN Convention on the Prohibition of Slavery in 1948. Slavery still exists in different countries today—the number of people in slavery is estimated to be almost twenty-five million. In one form or another, slavery exists in Sudan, Mauritania, Ghana, Thailand, China, Brazil, and many other countries. Human trafficking is a profitable business.

Colonies in North America:

French: Canada, modern Nova Scotia, New Brunswick, Louisiana, and Illinois.

Spanish colonies: Florida, California, and New Mexico.

Netherlands: Owned a colony in the state of New York.

COLONIZATION OF AMERICA

The discovery of America by Christopher Columbus allowed Spain to become the most significant colonial empire. A large part of South America spoke Spanish. Huge revenues from the new colonies filled the royal treasury. Numerous missionaries who poured into new colonies built temples, spread Christianity, and introduced the local population to the new faith. In North America, Spain owned California.

In the early seventeenth century, the British colonists obtained a license from King James I and founded a colony in Virginia. The primary income of the new colony was the production of tobacco. In May 1607, a fort named Jamestown was built in the Chesapeake Bay.

The beginning of colonization by England, the New World, was the arrival of the ship Mayflower with

102 Puritans Calvinists in September 1620. The colonists acquired a group of enslaved Africans. From this moment, the history of slavery in America begins. Here was one of the main reasons for the collapse of the future leader of the free world, but then no one could imagine a great future or the reasons for its collapse.

The first colony of New England was followed by numerous Puritan settlers who founded many settlements. Over the next quarter of a century, thirteen more colonies were formed. They were already representatives of different nationalities and beliefs. The colonies made great strides in the production of industrial goods and the construction of ships.

The metropolis wanted to see only a raw appendage in the colonies and forbade building ships. All goods were to be transported on British ships, and all goods for colonies should be shipped only from Britain. Dissatisfaction with the colonists' policy of the metropolis increasingly resulted in a desire to gain independence. Benjamin Franklin, in 1754, proposed a project to create a union of North American colonies with its government. This union was supposed to be led by the president appointed by the king of England. Such a project did not find support from the British Parliament.

The war between France and England (1754–1763), called the Seven Years' War, began in Europe and spread to the American Colonies. The military experience gained by militias who participated in the fighting was beneficial during the fight for independence. Colonists resented the new taxes in favor of the metropolis.

Constant skirmishes between the colonists and the royal military led to armed resistance. Members of Congress of the thirteen colonies gathered in Philadelphia in May 1775 and decided to mobilize the militias led by George Washington. The rebels captured Boston and retreated to New York.

In 1773, a group of daredevils infiltrated three British ships in Boston Harbor and threw 342 tea boxes overboard. This "Boston Tea Party," named so later, triggered repression, a ban on maritime trade, and legislative assemblies.

On July 4, 1776, deputies of the thirteen colonies adopted the Declaration of Independence. The colonies of Great Britain in North America announced they were creating an independent state—the United States of America.

On September 3, 1783, Britain recognized the independence of the United States. The War of Independence, what the American Revolution was called at the time, lasted from 1775 to 1783. Many European citizens were in the war on the side of the colonies against the British crown.

The victory of the colonial and now–independent states over the largest royal commonwealth had far-reaching consequences. The Declaration of Independence ushered in a new era of relations, becoming the first document in history to declare a free and independent state's legitimate natural rights. *All men have been created equal... the right to life, freedom, and the pursuit of happiness.*

All the states of Europe were under the rule of monarchs. The Declaration of Human Rights, the great French Revolution document, marked the beginning of all the following centuries' revolutionary movements.

The United States became the first state where a democratic majority of the population elected the government. The principles of statehood laid down by the Founding Fathers balanced many generations of relations between the government and the people's free choice.

At the time of the country's creation, July 4, 1776, Congress adopted the final text of the Declaration of Independence. It was proposed to condemn slavery but rejected by the majority. It was not considering the issues of slavery, which later pushed swung the pendulum, threatening to destroy the apparent equilibrium.

Thomas Jefferson, who chaired a five-member commission to draft the Declaration of Independence, included a section condemning slavery and the enslaving —people trade. This section was deleted at the request of South Carolina and Georgia representatives. Many of them were enslavers. The decision was to postpone the resolution of this issue for twenty years for the next generation. Perhaps this erroneous decision laid down a time bomb that would lead the country to disintegration sooner or later.

The world is forever divided between the past and the present.

Declared human equality for life, freedom, and the pursuit of happiness is an inalienable right of everyone. The country's population, by free vote, chose government representatives for a certain period. The dynastic despotism of power has been replaced by the will of free citizens, who choose the most worthy leaders from their midst.

The US Constitution was created on September 17, 1787, and ratified by nine states on June 21, 1788.

Subsequently, twenty-seven amendments were adopted to the Constitution, which ensured stability and prosperity for the country. The US Constitution's heart is the separation of executive, judicial, and legislative powers.

The Founding Fathers laid down several protective mechanisms that prevented the country from entering a political deadlock for many years. For almost a quarter of a millennium, the country had to supplement the Constitution twenty-seven times, introducing more amendments and ensuring its stability and prosperity.

There are many battered phrases and expressions used in certain life situations. The Jewish king, Solomon, is credited with a supposed phrase on his ring: *everything passes, and it will pass.* The following phrase is also attributed to King Solomon: nothing is *forever under the moon.*

The history of *Homo sapiens* and the events of the twenty-first century confirms these sayings of Solomon.

The Founding Fathers of the American Constitution tried to foresee any circumstances preventing a still very young state from making mistakes and creating upheavals. On the one hand, it was in danger of a dictatorship; on the other, one party's preponderance and the imbalance in the country's governance.

They divided the powers into legislative, executive, and judicial, preventing power concentration from one party's preponderance and imbalance in governing the country. The idea of checks and balances was thoroughly thought out and enshrined in the Constitution. The division of powers into legislative, executive, and judicial distributed responsibility among government branches, preventing power concentration by providing checks and balances. Democratic free elections for representatives of the legislative and executive branches guaranteed political freedom. Each branch had the right to test or restrict others from becoming the supreme power. The executive branch's changeability is utterly different from that of the Supreme Court. Those judges have lifetime tenure and can remain in their positions until they wish to retire voluntarily, making them independent and not under pressure.

The president of the United States is elected for a four-year term by popular vote.

The incumbent president may be re-elected for a second term. The head of the state's election is always accompanied by an escalation of the confrontation between the two main parties, democrats and republicans.

Such a confrontation is fraught with the danger of crisis for the country and possible widespread unrest. A body, a unique electoral college from each state, has been established to elect a president. The state's electoral votes are won by winning most of the votes in that state. The winner gets all.

The Senate and House of Representatives. Legislative power belongs to the bicameral Congress of the United States. This branch of government consists of state-elected representatives under a particular scheme. States elect their representatives to the legislative branch of government. Its members are limited in time but can be re-elected countless times. It depends only on those who live in a given state which candidate will be elected.

The Founding Fathers re-debated the constitutional formation of the legislature, which proceeded from the principle of democracy as a basis for determining the composition of Congress. Since the power source is the people, the composition of the US Congress's chambers depends on their choice.

The upper house of Congress— the Senate— consists of representatives (two senators from each state) elected for six years. Members of the lower House of Representatives (the number of representatives is proportional to each state's population, elected for two years, and six without the right to vote) are elected by the people. Most of all, the Founding Fathers were concerned about the possibility of concentrating power in one of the branches. Such an advantage could lead to dictatorship and tyranny.

Naturally, there were fears that the compromises found could lead to negative results. Society was still very young, and the Founding Fathers could not foresee the legislation's results. It could only be determined from the position of the past tense. It was a social formation, a unique experiment in the history of *Homo sapiens*.

The Constitution has allowed society to withstand and survive without much upheaval to the present day, and it is worthy of approval and admiration. The people who inhabited this country were pioneers. People wanted freedom for themselves and their children. They did not expect handouts from anyone. People mastered the land of this country and created its future. They knew they could only rely on themselves. The desire to create something of their own, equal opportunities for everyone, the labor invested, and the freedom of entrepreneurship have made it possible for this country's people to create a successful and happy life. It's a wonder how it happened; this country became the wealthiest country globally, the leader and guarantor of democratic freedoms and human rights, in a historically short period. The answer lies on the surface, although many do not want to believe it.

The entire population of our planet, *Homo sapiens*, has come the same way, but different ideologies, religions, and ways of development have led to different results. There are advanced modern countries with prosperous populations, democratic freedoms, a developed economy, and the opposite. Just look at South and North Korea, Saudi Arabia and Iran, modern Russia, and the countries of Eastern Europe. This series can be continued, but it is clear that ideologies or religions make some people happy or miserable.

The US has chosen its path. Enthusiasts built this unique country, immigrants seeking freedom, human rights, and the opportunity to build their destiny. They didn't expect help from anyone.

They were private entrepreneurs, sometimes putting their lives on the map, risking every minute to die from diseases, starvation, arrows of Indians, bullets of bandits, or wild predators' teeth. They had a chance, win or die. They, the entrepreneurs, built this country, which made them Americans.

They had no idea that in this country's well-being had been laid with timebombs that would destroy everything created for almost 250 years.

However, the problem of racial discrimination and slavery has not disappeared. Slavery was abolished in the United States in December 1865 after the end of the Civil War. The country's Black population's desegregation required considerable time, funds, particular decisions of the Supreme Court, and thousands of civil rights movements. Nothing goes without a trace. No good intentions, amendments to laws, prohibitions, and calls can instantly change the traditions developed over the centuries.

Racial problems have not gone away. In the twenty-first century, ethnic tensions are evident in many cities. Reversed racism appeared due to the segregation of the Black population, which still existed in the 1960s. The declared equality of races, genders, and minorities was perceived as a weakness of the white population. Handouts on preemptive rights when applying for a job or studying in higher education did not suit the Black population and other minorities.

They don't just want equality; they demand retribution for years of slavery and humiliation.

They demand from the white population not just an apology. They demand that this country be given to them because they believe that they've built that country, and a fair decision would be to redistribute the acquired economic wealth among those who created it.

This country is built on the blood and sweat of enslaved Black people, brought forcibly, shackled like wild animals—say the leaders of various black-skinned movements. Black people are much more likely than the rest of the population to end up behind bars. They are convinced that ordinary racism is behind this. In the United States, the black population makes up 12 to 14 percent of the total population, and the statistics of violent crimes committed by African Americans reach 50 percent.

The BLM, ANTIFA, and other such groups demand the abolition of the police as the primary solution to solve the problem. A movement to deprive police of funds gains unprecedented support.

BLM's co-founder explains why: "While we see that a lot of anger and outrage and frustration was sparked by the vicious murder of George Floyd, it's also clear to me that we have been sitting in our homes, navigating the pandemic, dealing with loved ones being sick, dealing with a great deal of fear and concern about what the day and the future will hold."

CAPITALISM

T he modern capitalist theory is traditionally traced to the eighteenth-century treatise *An Inquiry into the Nature and Causes of the Wealth of Nations* by Scottish political economist Adam Smith. The free–market economy came after feudalism as a logical system for production and distribution on the world market.

The development of capitalism was driven by the growth of the English cloth industry in the sixteenth, seventeenth, and eighteenth centuries. This development distinguishes capitalism from previous economic systems since capital accumulation made it possible to increase the necessary production capacities and produce mass products with the involvement of hired labor, with the distribution of surplus value created.

Wage labor turned out to be much more profitable

than bonded labor. There was an increase in labor productivity due to the production of more and more demanded goods. A new class emerged, workers. Lumpen, with nothing but working hands, ready to work for the minimum wage.

Capitalism requires working hands like any other form of social and economic goods production. Thousands of nonprofit businesses exist and thrive without the want of profit. But the natural goal of any business is to make a profit. Without such an incentive, a business cannot exist. Of course, such a community was divided into classes. The highest level was taken by people who had achieved significant success and earned significant capital. They were followed by managers of various levels, who received high remuneration and bonuses from the companies they worked for. Those who worked for hire were at the bottom of the social ladder.

Politicians, government officials, talented people in various fields of the arts, athletes who have achieved significant success, judges, lawyers, and many others employed were significant sectors of the country's economy.

As time passed, more and more immigrants came to the United States, hearing about extraordinary opportunities in this new *Promised Land*. Many people knew the degree of risk and the possibility of failure in an unfamiliar land in another community. Newcomers

risked everything they had in their abandoned homeland: relatives, friends, property, a well-established way
of life, and a particular societal position. All this was in
the past. Ahead was the unknown land, a different
language, a different way of life, and strangers. New
immigrants believed in their fortune and were ready
for any conditions, determined not to break but to find
their place on this earth.

Of course, there were adventurers, slackers, lazy
people, some with a criminal past, or just weak spirits
or unhealthy people. Society needed laws to protect
those who had failed to find a place in that country.
Free benefits have always attracted more people, and it
happened; they were selflessly helped without requiring
even gratitude in return. Masses of petitioners, who no
longer asked for but insisted on their rights specified in
the laws, reached the country.

The free allowances in social housing, food
coupons, medicine, education, and the pinnacle of
naive humanism, the advantages of rights in society's
social structure were given away for free, and more
people sought to take advantage of it.

In a socialist system, the cost of labor and benefits
are declared by law. Unfortunately, this doesn't work.
On the contrary, nothing corrupts more than receiving
demanded indulgences and preferences. Lack of moti-

vation to work at full strength leads to a natural desire to avoid unnecessary stress.

Since the benefits are required by law, it is unnecessary to make an effort to get up, work, and get less than one would get on benefits anyway. Entire neighborhoods, whole cities, are being created where people who receive benefits live. The environment already prepares children to accept such a way of life, not wanting to fight for their social life. Drugs, alcoholism, crime, and domestic violence make these ghettos a lousy environment to manage, even promising new indulgences and preferences. The white population of such districts is contemptuously called *white trash*.

Naturally, there are areas of poor populations, people living on benefits. The majority of the population of such areas comprises different minorities. With the right to vote, such an environment instinctively chooses the worst, most evil, and hypocritical politicians who indulge such communities' desires.

These low-income communities provide an ideal environment for representatives of the US Democratic Party. Thomas Jefferson founded the oldest party in the country. In the mid-twentieth century, the party began to noticeably shift to the left in the political palette, uniting the social-liberal and social-democratic ideologies of helping disadvantaged and vulnerable voters.

The Democratic Party favors increasing social spending, raising taxes on the wealthy and large corporations, fighting pollution, supporting any minority, family planning, and restricting the freedom to sell weapons in the United States.

Democrats unite socially liberal and democratic ideologies to help low-income and vulnerable groups. Various minorities loudly demand respect for their rights.

Victorious demonstrations of all kinds of minorities demanding the right and freedom to express their views and changes in social and constitutional laws. The bill was no longer for thousands but millions of new citizens. Among them are feminist, ethnic, racial, nationalistic, and religious groups. Both legal and illegal immigration to the United States has grown.

The notorious melting pot was puffing at full steam, in naive confidence to melt into a single monolithic nation, ready to work hard and create the dream of humanity—a paradise of equal opportunities for every individual.

Theoretically, it was a brilliant idea. The problem was the very nature of *Homo sapiens.* Since the first center of civilization's construction more than five thousand years ago, this species has been divided into classes. Some commanded while others obeyed orders. So it was also during the communal primitive society.

Dominant, cruel leaders commanded and punished those who did not show due respect or please the leader. As a species of great apes, we belong to one of the cruelest families of animals. Humans have lost their ferocity, but our ancestors' limbic system can prevail in particular circumstances, such as during puberty. It is accompanied by physiological and mental changes in the human body, forcing us to obey the instinct of reproduction.

From creating the first civilization to the present day, human history has been marked by bloody wars, enslavement, extreme cruelty, and intolerance.

The twentieth century brought two bloody world wars and even more bloody civil confrontations, set on fire by Marxist revolutionaries, enthusiastically met with society's left-centrist mood. Europe, trying not to concede to America in liberalism, opened its doors to refugees from the Middle East and Africa.

The population's demographics have changed dramatically over a quarter of a millennium. Democracy has become the ideology/religion.

Democrats moved far left on the political spectrum and have become neo-democrats, too radical, and close to the socialists in their vision of rebuilding the world. It would seem that the ideas of Marxism were tested in different countries: —Russia, China, North Korea, Vietnam, Cuba, and Venezuela—proved not viability but rather a dangerous slide to totalitarianism, destruction of any freedoms, and disintegration of the economy. But people learned nothing and craved power to repeat the failed socialist idea.

Thomas Jefferson warned, "Democracy will cease

to exist when you take away from those willing to work and give to those who wouldn't."

Respect for democratic freedoms may be threatened by the concentration in the legislature of representatives willing to submit to the demands of the unstable masses of society.

Twenty-First
Century—
Confrontation

*H*omo *sapiens* invented weapons of mass destruction and deadly viruses that can destroy all living things. The perceived danger of our species' very existence and the consequences of the devastating world wars of the twentieth century led to the creation of the United Nations, which replaced the League of Nations, created after World War I. This international organization is designed to prevent bloody upheaval and help those unable to cope with their problems because of the circumstances. As it did happen many times in history, such organizations are becoming feeders for politicians and tools of pressure on the organizations involved in financing.

Countries and continents are still torn apart by contradictions, and peace on our planet can explode at the whim or wild ambition of any ruler wielding weapons of mass destruction. The twenty-first century may be the most monstrous and perhaps the most destructive to the species *Homo sapiens*. Possibly destroying the whole planet. What is the reason for such a pessimistic forecast? There are many of them, and we will consider everything in order.

The year 2020 could be remembered for generations as the coronavirus pandemic that has shaken practically the entire world's population. However, it cannot be compared to the early twentieth century's pandemic, the "Spanish flu" that claimed more than fifty million lives in two years. The upheaval in the world economy and the number of countries covered by the short-term COVID-19 pandemic showed to the naive mind of *Homo sapiens* how ephemeral its protection is against the challenges of nature, probable human error, or targeted military development. The unexpected pandemic has demonstrated the fragile lives of everyone and the world's population.

By mid-2020, the total number of people infected had grown to 22.4 million, with 788,000 dead. The most alarming circumstance was that scientists had not yet prepared a vaccine to prevent infection and effective treatment for a newly-discovered virus that can spread almost instantly across countries and continents. Everything that could be closed was closed. The Earth's population wore masks and disinfected everything that could be disinfected. All countries have gone into deep quarantine, leaving a minimum of stores selling food and pharmacies, which the world's population cannot do without. Such drastic measures have probably paid off the expected results but have caused side effects that may be worse than the pandemic. The destruction of economies in almost all countries ruined and bankrupted small entrepreneurs and the economy's giants.

Financial support from the governments of rich countries that give people printed money cannot solve the population's problems, making them unsure of where and how they will live tomorrow. Businesses are forced to lay off hundreds of thousands, if not millions, of employees worldwide and close their doors forever. Many areas of the population's activities became unnecessary, without which modern humans could not imagine how to cope.

Urbanization—urban population growth—is due to people searching for better living conditions and improving their children's futures. More than half of the world's population lives in cities. In today's digital economy, cities are the ideal place to live comfortably.

Advantages include work, urban transport, water and sewerage systems infrastructure, health care, renting or purchasing housing with multi-year installment payments, schools, and children's institutions. All this is connected with modern humans' desire to enjoy life, spend idle time in bars, restaurants, shopping malls, shops, theaters, or walk on beautifully lit streets with elegant, carefree people.

All these benefits of civilization make life in cities attractive. There is always an opportunity to find a new, more attractive, and better-paid job in urban life. Sometimes there were severe economic disasters. Employers went bankrupt and fired everyone who worked for the firm. People have to find a new home or learn another profession.

Social conditions guarantee unemployment benefits for a certain period or help them enter a new profession, have allowed them to survive temporary difficulties. It is possible to open a small family business in urban environments and not hire workers in the beginning. Work hard and long hours, survive temporary difficulties. Having a four-door car can be engaged legally or illegally in private haulage. The main thing is to have a desire and not to give up. Not to be afraid of any, even the dirtiest and most unprestigious work. The city always needs working hands.

Simultaneously, city governments' social benefits have always attracted people who have used various tricks to obtain many benefits. Social housing is available for people experiencing poverty, benefits the individual, and assistance from virtuous public funds and influential politicians betting on such population segments. Government agencies have special funds to support those unable or who do not want to fit into society's generally accepted residence rules.

Cities have always attracted illegal businesses. Unstable, dependent, oppressed people, or those who have inherited pathologies from their parents, are addicted and are willing to commit any crime to get the desired dose of drugs.

Addiction and substance abuse lead to the destruction of the body and dementia. The drug mafia is the most extensive crime, earning billions on downtrodden people's addictions.

In the cities, areas are formed of decayed, mentally ill people living on the streets and not want to settle in places created by the city administration for homeless people. They feed themselves on donations or wait for philanthropic or urban groups to deliver lunches in places where the homeless and drug addicts are crowded. Among such population groups are infirm people of old age, sick people suffering from various physical or mental ailments, and chronic diseases. Many countries previously had laws that qualified vagrancy and begging as illegal and asocial. Reluctance to work, vagrancy, and living in public places, parks, and public transport were considered a violation of the established order and could lead to a penalty of imprisonment. In the enlightened liberal twentieth century, such a way of life is not challenged or condemned. Citizens are required to respect the rights of free human beings.

The urban population was the most affected by the coronavirus pandemic. Closed businesses and offices have splashed out on the streets; millions of people who built their lives on the opportunities to work and earn enough to provide a certain standard of living and ensure old age.

Entrepreneurs in services, tourism, food, entertainment, and related businesses have suffered economic losses due to the pandemic. Those whose income depended on the volume of goods or services provided closed simultaneously. There is no loophole or opportunity to use their talents or knowledge. Any mass entertainment or sporting events are prohibited. Survivors included those who stayed at home and could work remotely using a computer.

Almost all countries declared a quarantine and a ban on leaving or entering the country. This decision undermined the foundations of the economy but seemed to save the population. The experience of the previous pandemic, the "Spanish flu," at the beginning of the twentieth century showed that the population's salvation positively impacted economic recovery.

The world collapsed. The social situation created by generations had melted away, taking away confidence in the future. The real threat of homelessness, inability to pay loans, families' destruction, bankruptcy, and impotent despair came with the loss of work or business. Lost hope for a secure old age, stability of the habitual way of life, savings—the habit of living on loan, when credit seemed to solve all social and vital problems.

The fear of children's unknown future and the real threat of becoming another victim of the deadly virus pushed people to protest against the authorities, which gave financial handouts and assurances to resolve the situation shortly.

The problem was not in power. Natural disasters and wars have always happened at least every hundred years. In a local natural disaster, all the country's forces were mobilized to deal with the consequences and help those affected. In war, an enemy must be defeated at all costs by enormous efforts and casualties among the population. This pandemic has hit all countries and continents at the same time. No one in the world has been prepared for such a challenge. There was no cure or treatment and no vaccine for immunity against infection.

All the medical science on earth cannot create a cure or vaccine tomorrow. It takes time and long trials on living people. Sooner or later, scientists will be able to find ways to fight this new virus. Was it human-made or natural? There was no alternative. Survive or die. Humanity has experienced black pox, cholera, bubonic plague, Spanish flu, syphilis, tuberculosis, and many other contagious diseases that have taken millions of lives. *Homo sapiens* survived. There is hope to survive as well in this time.

SLAVERY IN THE UNITED STATES

E nslaved people trade has flourished in America since its starting point in 1619. Norfolk and New Orleans were important national enslaved people markets, as well as Charleston, South Carolina. By 1860, there were four million enslaved people in the United States.

The enslaved people's labor brought from Africa was widely used on many plantations growing tobacco, coffee, corn, rice, sugar cane, cotton, vegetables, and animal husbandry. In the United States, most enslaved people were Black Africans forcibly removed by enslaved-people traders from the African continent. The English colonists brought the first enslaved people to Virginia in 1619. The English Parliament in 1698 legalized the enslaved people's trade for individuals.

The Civil War was preceded by a movement of white Protestants of the North, who advocated abolishing slavery. Protestants proclaimed the idea of slavery contrary to the Bible. This Civil War of 1861–1865 is also called the war of the North and the South. The causes of the war lay in the economic sphere. In the country's North were various industrial enterprises employed by immigrants from different countries.

The northern states needed raw materials, especially cotton. The southern states owned huge fertile plantations that employed black-skinned enslaved people from Africa. The planters wanted to sell their goods in Europe, where raw material prices were much higher.

The main disagreement was related to the further development of the country. Southerners wanted freedom and independence from the supreme power country's government. The Northerners sought to subjugate all the central government states under the enforcement of laws. The US annexed more territories and raised questions about each new state's constitution and whether enslaved people were owned or were free.

The Republican Party, formed in 1854, was led by the country's president in 1860, Abraham Lincoln, a staunch opponent of slavery. Southern states voted to withdraw from the Union and formed the Confederate States of America. Lincoln declared the southern states rebels and encouraged volunteers to join the army. The Civil War on land and at sea was fought with varying success.

On December 30, 1862, Lincoln signed the *Emancipation Proclamation on the Liberation of Enslaved People.* The war finally defined the purpose of the northerners, the abolition of slavery.

By 1865, the Confederate Army was surrounded by the Union Army under General Grant's command. General Lee won several brilliant victories and intended to break the northerners in a decisive final battle.

The Northerners won a significant victory at Gettysburg in July 1863. This war was the bloodiest in the history of the United States. More than 620 000 people on both sides were killed outright or died later from wounds.

The prohibition of slavery was enshrined in the Thirteenth Amendment to the US Constitution.

With the release of many enslaved people, the question arose of what to do with this population. The American Colonization Society, founded in 1816, supported free African Americans who decided to return to Africa. The society helped establish a colony in Liberia. Supporters of the resettlement of formerly enslaved Americans included abolitionists and some enslavers who wanted to get rid of the formerly enslaved people. They were aware of the potential threat to the foundations of the existing society. They believed that Black people would have many opportunities and a more supportive environment in Africa than in America. Thousands of African American free citizens moved from America to Liberia.

With the end of the Civil War and the abolition of slavery, the number of free African Americans has grown significantly. Many saw the solution to this challenging problem in emigration. The US Congress allocated $100000 for the organization ACS (assistance to African Americans who decided to move to Liberia). The legislatures of several states also allocated money. The society existed for many years, but the idea of resettlement to Africa did not support most of the country's African American population.

In July 1868, the Fourteenth Amendment to the US Constitution was enacted, granting citizenship to anyone born in the United States. That automatically proclaimed the equality of all citizens of the country, regardless of skin color.

Nevertheless, segregation existed in separate education, demarcated public transport, public places (cafes, restaurants), military units, etc.

The US Supreme Court ruled 1954 that racial segregation should be legally banned. Democratic president John F. Kennedy proposed the Civil Rights Act. After his assassination in November 1963, the new president, Lyndon B. Johnson, introduced the law. The US House of Representatives passed the bill on February 10, 1964. President Johnson signed the Civil Rights Act on July 2, 1964.

In 1964, the Twenty-Fourth Amendment to the Constitution was adopted, prohibiting discrimination based on race, color, religion, sex, national origin, and sexual orientation. This amendment allowed every citizen of the country to vote, regardless of whether the person paid taxes or not. The Voting Rights Act of 1965 abolished most voting requirements other than citizenship.

CONSEQUENCES OF SLAVERY

Centuries of slavery and centuries-old colonial politics have cultivated the fruits of social-communist thinking among many of society's segments. Conquering countries and continents, the colonizers brought civilization in the form of robbery from indigenous peoples, slavery, and the forcible imposition of religious beliefs on the population living there. Naturally, all this caused resistance to the colonialists. They responded by destroying all those who disagreed with the dictates of the new masters. Whole civilizations and nationalities disappeared, and the rest adopted the values of the Christian world.

The colonizers' countries were flooded with valuables, among which gold and silver stood out. Minting such a mass of gold and silver coins breathed in a new economic jet, which allowed the creation of new types of spheres of production. In the British Empire of the fifteenth and sixteenth centuries, there was an agricultural revolution, which eventually led to the Industrial Revolution. Farmers were introduced to new agricultural machinery, using steam engines and plows, improving drainage work with new equipment.

The development of agriculture stimulated the creation of industry. Demand for the products needed to wage wars provided the market. New technological capabilities, machines, and mechanisms brought the cotton industry to a new level. The steam engine was widely used in various industries, including engineering, coal, machine-building, shipbuilding, and vehicle manufacturing. Many new factories created the conditions for the emergence of the Industrial Revolution.

These required significant investments, intensive labor, and the availability of a market to consume manufactured products. The Industrial Revolution led to a change in the class composition of the population. Industrial cities created housing complexes, more like slums for the poor. The mechanization of production reduced jobs and significantly reduced wages. Urbanization made most of the population poor wage-dependent workers—the loss of the ability to work led to poverty. All these conditions led to the creation of various strike movements and resistance. Marxism did not appear suddenly. It was preceded by various utopian theories of the world's reconstruction, which speak about the world's fairness and equality of all who relate to sentient beings. Marx's theory of armed seizure of power pointed to the practical ways Marxist followers took advantage. Revolutions happened before the advent of Marxism.

The absolute dynastic monarchy was outdated and inevitably had to be replaced by a new form of government.

The Dutch Revolution of the sixteenth and seventeenth centuries against Spanish rule led to Europe's first bourgeois republic.

The English Revolution of 1640–1688 restricted the monarch's rights.

The American Revolution of 1775–1783 created the Declaration of Independence of the United States.

The Great French Revolution of 1789 gave birth to the Declaration of Human Rights.

In France in 1830, a new revolution changed the dynasty.

The European Revolutions of 1848 swept many European countries—Italy, German states, Austria, Romania, and Prussia. The monarchy gave way to republics, where new constitutions were adopted.

In Russia, the first revolution took place in 1905. The people got freedom of speech and elections.

The February Revolution took place in Russia in 1917. In October, Marxists led by Ulyanov-Lenin seized power in the country.

We know from history how all these revolutions ended. In 1918, there were revolutions in Germany and Austria. The Great French and Russian Bolshevik revolutions ended in bloody bacchanalia and terror. The German Weimar Republic brought the bloodiest tyrant in history—Adolf Hitler. The rest of the European revolutions brought constitutional freedoms and civil rights to their people.

US Election 2020

I n 2020, the US faced a revolutionary situation, ready to destroy the country's constitutional stability, which allowed this country to become the free world leader, the guarantor of democratic freedoms and equality of citizens of this country. The system established by the Founding Fathers and the US Constitution kept this country from turmoil and revolution. The main concern of those who founded this country was to prevent a slide into tyranny by concentrating all power in the hands of one branch of government. Periodic election, delimitation of powers, and the president's limitation to two four-year terms of office guaranteed legal continuity. Democratic presidential and congressional elections have stabilized the system for more than a quarter of a millennium.

As it turns out, the system is out of date. The system was not responding to the side effects of this country's history and demographic changes—such a diverse society, where some consider themselves infringed on their rights and require special treatment.

Various minorities demand advantages, where the ideologies of building society are directly opposite and irreconcilable. Such a society is not viable but is ready to defend its ideas at any cost, up to armed resistance.

History has shown that irreconcilable confrontation leads to civil war. The northern states versus the Confederacy led to the Civil War of 1861–1865. The socioeconomic systems in opposing groups of states became the causes of the war. The bourgeois North opposed the enslaved people–owning South. Slavery was declared to be the leading cause of the war. The bloodiest confrontation in the history of the United States did not teach our species, *Homo sapiens*.

Today, in 2021, the US is again split into two almost equal halves. On the one hand, people who are adherents of traditional American values. It's the American dream: freedom, owning a home, bank account, confidence in the future—justice of all before the law, and the opportunity to succeed in life.

The other half of the country, passionate about socialist equality ideas, demands wealth be taken from the rich and divided among those who have failed to succeed with their work. Using the discontent of many population segments blaming their failures on the wealthy, neo-democrats promise a significant increase in taxes on the successful, distributing significant funds among the poorest.

Modern liberal ideas are trendy today in American society.

In academia, the ideas of civil liberties are the dominant ideology, especially among social and humanities teachers. There are demands to increase social security for the population, free medicine, free higher education, and environmental protection. The neo-democrats believe that the government should solve all social problems by caring for society's economic life's poorest segments. According to the neo-democrats, high taxes and liberal legislation will allow the government to manage and distribute income, maintaining the financial balance in the country.

That's how all the revolutions known to us began. These naive and perverse ideas were embedded in gullible supporters' heads, ready to overthrow and destroy the old "unjust" order. Taking away and dividing is passable if one is not afraid to stain one's hands in the blood of those who built and created the country's wealth. Of course, there will be sacrifices, economic losses, and the destruction of moral and material values. Giving up principles and morality is possible for a bright and radiant future. But the main question remains, will everyone be equal and happy in this "beautiful" future?

Naive humanity has forgotten its past—the species

Homo sapiens stores in its brain the instincts inherent in our species' biological nature. Our instincts dictate our motives for behavior. We strive to create and multiply values, provided that close people, family, and those we love can use what we have created in this life. When we have gone, we want to know that those we love will remember us with gratitude.

The idea of creating, taking risks, and working hard is unimaginable to a person with an enslaved person mentality. Forced submission is incapable of creating. It is possible to take and distribute, but to create, knowing that what has been created will be taken away, is hardly possible. All the revolutions collapsed about this simple notion: mine, my family, my piece of bread. The economy is a harsh teacher.

The Great French and Socialist Russian Revolutions destroyed their countries' economies and moved to their associates' cruel terror and destruction, trying to shift the responsibility for their stupidity. What is happening before our eyes in America today is, in fact, a revolution. It happened in a non-standard way. Here, the lower classes did not storm the White House. Neo-democrats took advantage of loopholes in the country's outdated constitution through rigged elections, seized power, and subjugated and intimidated all who prevented establishing a new order.

All government branches, the presidency, Congress (both chambers), Supreme Court, power structures, armies, media, and social networks are ready to cooperate and help the new government. This almost bloodless revolution occurred because society was prepared for it by promoting hatred of the existing capitalist social system. The tempting utopian idea of universal equality turned out to be so attractive that the naive species of *Homo sapiens* forgot history. However, many did not even know our species' history and followed the preachers' dream of absolute happiness.

What happened in the US in 2020 was supposed to happen in 2016. Hillary Clinton was the only leading Democratic nominee. The media unanimously predicted her victory as the logical follower of society's democratization, gloriously started by the Clintons and continued by the Obama administration. Unexpectedly for everyone and therefore incredibly unpleasant for the Democrats, it was not a politician who came to power, but a Republican businessman, Donald Trump. The Neo-Democratic Party was about to celebrate the landmark tradition of the sixteen years' Clinton-Obama administration.

Over the years, the Democratic Party has changed dramatically, moving even further to the far left on the political spectrum. A new young radical change came to the party.

There are still quite brave, experienced fighters in

battles for power, like Nancy Pelosi, Chuck Schumer, and many others. But younger and more radical newcomers already set the party's tone. First elected to the lower house of Congress, they loudly stated their demands and vision for the future of the Democratic Party, led by this new vision of the country's future radical four, which received the nickname *"Squad"* according to the American tradition.

This group of radicals is headed by AOC (Alexandra Ocasio-Cortez). They demand radical change. They demand even radical changes in the country's foreign and domestic policy. Incumbent President Donald Trump has sharply disliked this group, and they insist on his removal from power in any way available.

It might seem that this is just a tribute to the radicalism of youth inherent in puberty and raging hormones, but this young squad demanded their place at the party's helm. Soon enough, it became clear that behind them was a considerable part, mainly of the country's young and radical population. Naturally, numerous minorities of all colors of the rainbow demanded radical changes.

All four years of Donald Trump's presidency have passed in the struggle for survival—slander, media harassment of Trump's actions, and his family.

He steadfastly and courageously endured all the blows and pursued a policy that brought the country an unprecedented economic rise. The coronavirus pandemic that hit the world in 2019, called *COVID-19*, demanded from the president nonstandard solutions and the creation of forces capable of resisting a devastating pandemic on a scale comparable to the famous Spanish flu of 1918–1920. Several pharmaceutical companies have created a vaccine that can quickly prevent the further spread of the COVID-19 virus. The year 2020, was accompanied by the unrest of thousands of protesters against the government. The organized gangs of young men, who resembled the brown-shirt groups of fascist Germany, attested to actual pogroms and toppled the statues—crowds of looters smashed shop windows and plundered businesses.

The masses, instigated by the emerging leaders, clashed with the police, burned police cars, and demanded deprivation of the last budget funds or elimination of police. In states ruled by Democrats, police officers were required not to interfere with "peaceful protesters."

The riots, arson, looting, and demands that the white population kneel in front of the black population and kiss their feet or shoes, thus expressing remorse for the suffering caused by the enslavers, all took place in the middle of the day on the crowded streets of cities. In New York City, Mayor De Blasio, yielding to the "defund police" demands, cut the police budget by one billion dollars and went out with the protesters to paint the pavement in front of the building belonging to

President Donald Trump. On the pavement, a monumental inscription appeared many meters long: BLACK LIVES MATTER.

Police officers everywhere in the country and members of the lower house of Congress, led by Speaker Nancy Pelosi, knelt and signed off a request for forgiveness.

Leaders of the black population of the United States, BLM, and ANTIFA, demanded payments to all black people of the country "for reparations for all the years of slavery." BLM leader stated: "If we do not get everything we demand, we will burn this order."

The Democrats supported these demands.

The country's forty-sixth general election was held in a tradition on the first Tuesday of November, the third.

The GOP ran the forty-fifth president of the United States, Donald Trump. Democratic vice president in the administration of Barack Obama, Joe Biden, was running for the Democratic Party.

Long before the deadline, pre-voting polling stations were opened throughout the country. Unlike in previous years, those wishing to vote early lined up in huge queues. Democrats demanded an increase in the timing of the postal vote.

The vote was in full swing, and the nation's postal service could not cope with the massive flow of incoming ballots; President Donald Trump had spoken out against extending the postal vote. In violation of the Constitution, individual states independently decided to increase mail delivery, abandoning the standard conditions of the postal envelopes being stamped by mail on voting day.

The whole country was preparing for the elections. The state administration prepared polling stations and purchased state-of-the-art computer counting equipment. Both parties sent their representatives to organize checks at polling stations to prevent voting-rights violations and electoral fraud.

America had not known such a mass turnout of those wishing to vote for their candidate. Traditional liberal media and social media were reporting from all over the country. The polling stations closed at 8 p.m. local time, and votes were counted. The country did not sleep and followed the progress of the reports. President Donald Trump won traditionally pro-Republican states, and Joe Biden in pro-Democratic states. President Donald Trump was clearly in the lead in the race. Such proportion in voting continued until 3 a.m. Suddenly everything stopped.

Some failures were explained in the mechanical counting of votes with the purchased equipment. An hour and a half later, the counting process resumed, but with a fantastic result. Now in the lead was Barack Obama's vice president, Joe Biden. In America, there are so-called *wavering states* where votes can be given to one or another candidate. It was in these states that the voting results were decided. Joe Biden won.

The US has a system *of indirect elections* in which electors represent each state. Depending on its population, each state puts out a certain number of electoral votes. For example, California, the largest state, has fifty-five electoral votes, while Alaska's sparsely populated state has three electoral votes. Traditionally, all electoral votes for a state go to the candidate with the most votes. The winner is the candidate who receives at least 270 out of 538 electoral votes.

Simultaneously, with the president's election in 2020, elections for the US Congress, the Senate, and the House of Representatives were held this year.

The country's forty-fifth president will be known on December 14, 2020, when the Electoral College votes will be counted.

Scandals around the elections grew louder as the election date approached on November 3. An article accused Joe Biden of corruption in the New York Post in mid-October. It published a letter from the Ukrainian company Burisma to Biden's son; Hunter got gratitude for the organized meeting with Biden Sr. and asked him to use his influence to help the company.

Joe Biden claimed he had nothing to do with his son's work for Burisma.

Fox News Channel 5 showed a tape in which Barack Obama's vice president, Joe Biden, demanded that Ukrainian authorities remove Attorney General Shokhin, who was investigating Burisma, threatening otherwise to shut down $1.5 billion aid to Ukraine. Joe Biden has spent more than half a century in politics. He was vice president for eight years in the Obama administration.

Joe Biden was called, in his words, the "poorest man in Congress." Officially, from 1998 to 2019, the Biden family earned $22.5 million. Joe Biden's son, Hunter Biden, has been embroiled in several scandals. Corruption, sexual drug-related behavior, and receiving bribes from different countries.

Hunter Biden was hired on the scandalous Ukrainian energy company's board of directors, Burisma, for almost $1 million annually. In his letter, the company's management adviser "thanked Hunter for meeting with Biden, the vice president," and asked him to consider how he "could use his influence" to help the company.

Hunter Biden left his notebook in the repair shop but forgot to return for it. Rudy Giuliani, the former mayor of New York, a personal lawyer for President Trump, who got a copy of the hard disc from this note-book of Hunter Biden, said that he found "numerous photos; of minor age girls."

All materials were handed over to the police. Joe Biden has denied having anything to do with his son's work at Burisma.

The Justice Department drew attention to Hunter Biden's relationship with China. "Suspicious foreign transactions" and money from China and other countries are being *investigated*. President Donald Trump said, "Hunter received millions of dollars from Ukraine and China."

Former New York mayor Rudy Giuliani, Trump's lawyer, has claimed that Joe Biden used his son to receive bribes as a "gathering...a man to collect bribes."

He said another Hunter Biden hard drive was found in Boston. It contains "substantial evidence of bribery, espionage, money laundering" from different countries.

The son of a democratic politician allegedly received $1.5 million from the Chinese authorities and about $3 million from Ukraine.

"Yesterday, I learned that the US Attorney's office in Delaware informed my legal advisers of an investigation into my tax cases," Hunter Biden wrote in an open statement.

In 2017, when Joe Biden ended his time as vice president, his son helped CEFC China Energy strike a deal to invest in US energy projects.

A valuable gift attracted lawyers' attention; after one of the business meetings in 2017, the founder and former chairman of CEFC China Energy, Ye Jianming, presented Hunter Biden with a 2.8-carat diamond.

On questions to Joe Biden, then a presidential

candidate, about his son Hunter Biden's corruption ties, the answer was concise: "A slanderous company... As soon as I become president, I'll stop it."

Biden also said he "didn't get a penny" from foreign governments. The Democratic Party candidate reacted to Trump's accusations that he received $3.5 million from Russia and had a percentage of his son Hunter's business in Ukraine and China.

Kim Strassel, a member of The Wall Street Journal editorial board, said:

We have text messages and emails where all these partners say, "We should leave more money for the people who really work." It's not Hunter, by the way. "We should... What's Hunter's contribution?" and then Hunter violently intervenes; he says,

"You don't understand? I am the bargain. People do it just because they need Biden's name. It's my family's legacy."

American political turmoil continued until November 3, 2020, Election Day. Many predicted that "Trump well turned out" and expressed their opinions on what would happen on this critical day for the world. There were some variants.

The situation is unpredictable. Suppose Biden wins and Congress is under the control of the Democratic Party. In that case, the turmoil will probably subside quickly, and the country will predictably roll to the point of no return—it will turn into a left-wing-radical socialist state. The problem lies in deciding what to do with the vast, organized army of Black people, BLM, Antifa, and other groups that have democrats engage in big politics to counter President Trump and intimidate his supporters. Armed and organized groups that do not submit to a single command will not disappear and will not dissolve suddenly, allowing the democrats to enjoy the fruits of victory. They will demand their share, and the price may be much higher than democrats are willing to pay.

Over the next four years, a fierce struggle will take place between the radical left, the Democratic Party, and the conservative Republican Party. This struggle will most likely, albeit more slowly, lead to the option of continuing a permanent war between the president and the House of Representatives. If Trump wins but the House of Representatives stays with the Democratic Party, there will be a surge of turmoil and a spike in crime that will last two months, and then Trump will extinguish the unrest by force.

Trump will have his hands free, and with Senate backing, he may be able to halt or even reverse the country's degradation for at least the next four years.

There is another possible line of development of events. BLM, ANTIFA, and similar radical structures supporting the guilt of the living white population for centuries of slavery and the humiliation of the black-skinned people will require the allocation of territories to create their separate state territory of the United States. Compensation for centuries of slavery and humiliation establishes the newly formed state's boundaries. Have its regular army, weapons to guard the borders, currency, and laws that assert the inalienable right to create such a state on the United States territory. They are already trying this idea for strength. Leaders of such movements understand the benefits to be derived from such circumstances. Trillions of dollars in handouts won't satisfy them. Power and the ability to realize the most unthinkable uncontrollable desires are more substantial than drugs. And trillions of dollars will be brought in on a golden platter. Nothing corrupts like the lust for power. Humanity has gone through bloody stories of power struggles more than once. Consciousness poisoned by the slavery past, confidence in the existing infringement of the rights of the Black minority, and a sense of rejection in society demand action. Having tried their strength with impunity, they realized that they could win. For the past sixty to seventy years, the democratic public has indulged all the demands of various radical minorities and communities. Such a development will inevitably lead to a new civil war with dire consequences. Did democratic leaders calculate such similar scenarios? Whether they've prepared for that, we'll know if any events happen.

President Joe Biden and Vice President Kamala

Harris are ready to control this country. Controlling Congress by Democratic Party gave them much leverage. Multiple laws are passed following the vision of the neo-democrats. They are raising taxes and banning the free sale of weapons.

Return to all agreements made under Barack Obama's administration. The country's population must surrender the available weapons for a nominal fee, or a law obliging them to surrender weapons will be adopted. Censorship of all media, including social networks, is being introduced. Laws protecting the rights of minorities and providing preferential qualifications for employment in educational institutions and public offices are adopted. There are also advantages in tenders for any business activity and free health insurance for everyone. They will be restoring a transgender policy that includes men's access to women's locker rooms. There are also open borders and amnesty for all illegal immigrants with the right to vote.

They will be changing laws in the country's electoral system, giving them a lasting advantage in all future US elections—restoring all programs related to globalists and environmentalists—reparations to those who have suffered during slavery, segregation, and injustices in this country.

Many global corporations, which helped the

Democratic Party win, are waiting for their share in the carve-up of corporations associated with military equipment production, pharmaceutical giants, and industrialists whom Trump forced to return their products to the United States. Many others have suffered from Trump's policies. An enormous pie called the United States will change its name to the USSA-United Socialist States of America.

The Democratic Party will be forced to enact harsh measures to preserve the existing order and maintain its dominance. It is the logic of all revolutions. Meeting opposition, the ruling party will abolish all democratic freedoms: speech, assembly, change of power, respect for human rights, and the right to own weapons. All those who oppose the ruling party's decisions are declared enemies of the people, internal terrorists with all the ensuing consequences.

The history of *Homo sapiens* is known to have similar coups (palace or revolutionary). The losing party is declared an enemy of the people (country) and is persecuted, and terror accompanies slander. During the French Revolution, the case in Nazi Germany in the 1930s, and the Socialist Revolution in Russia, such upheavals have resulted in multiple casualties, famine, and economic disintegration in each country. It could be dangerous to separate those who disagree with such conditions of a particular scenario from the United

States. All states have the right to regulate various issues and powers where there may be a question of secession from the Union.

Such attempts to break away from the Union are fraught with violence, destruction of the country, and substantial population victims. Whether the US is insured against such a scenario will tell with time.

Today we know that the democrats won, and Joe Biden became the forty-sixth president of the United States.

PRESIDENT DONALD TRUMP

The president's opponents challenged the White House administration's achievements under President Donald Trump from 2017 to 2021. Why is such a harsh confrontation against him like a brutal war? The November 3, 2020, election drew a sharp line between his supporters and opponents. Half of the country considers President Donald Trump, the greatest president since Abraham Lincoln. The other half considers Trump the worst president since his first election day. They were hoping for his removal without hesitations, even in the impeachment process. From the beginning of his term, Trump said he would run for a second term. It's already beyond common sense. A vote in the November 3 election showed that nearly seventy-five million voters had voted for the president. It is a complete record, even more so for a president running for a second term. Joe

Biden, Trump's rival and former vice president in Obama's administration, won more than eighty-two million votes. The country's presidential contender lost out to his democratic rivals in a race in primary elections in all states.

In competition with President Donald Trump, the former vice-president of the government of Barack Obama, Joe Biden rarely appeared in front of the voters, hiding, as evil tongues claimed, in a shelter. So suddenly and unexpectedly, Biden pulled ahead and became the leader. Suddenly he overtook the record holder President Donald Trump, trendy among voters, by seven million votes.

The Democratic Party and the media declared Joe Biden's team president-elect (elected), with Kamala Harris as vice president, without waiting for congressional approval to be announced.

The media was filled with rumors and stories about unprecedented election fraud in the history of the United States, using modern technological means to count and (correct if necessary) in favor of (the desired candidate). We must treat all these publications and statements with caution, evaluating critically, expressed in the heat of a political battle. All further narration is based on the publications that appeared in the media.

There was apparent forgery and voter fraud. Trump's lawyer, former New York City Mayor Rudy Giuliani, said, "Do you think we're stupid?" Trump did not admit defeat in the election and decided to challenge the election results in court.

There was a massive amount of work to verify the election materials, process, and search for evidence of falsifications. The documents for filing and the court were prepared. Masses of documents, official affidavits, evidence of irregularities during the vote count, and surveillance footage need to be prepared. All work needed to be done since a two-stage election system, on November 14, the lists of electors from each state would be certified, and they, in turn, cast votes in favor of one or another candidate.

A team of lawyers led by Rudy Giuliani was formed to collect evidence of fraud in the 2020 US presidential election.

The state winner receives all electoral votes. It is enough to collect 270 electoral votes to win the presidential elections.

The president's legal team focused on vetting the so-called "swing" states. No clear majority of one party decided the election outcome: Pennsylvania, North Carolina, Ohio, Georgia, Wisconsin, Michigan, Nevada, and Iowa.

Many political experts have argued that Joe Biden's victory is a *fait accompli*. Some doubters believed that the US Supreme Court, dominated by Donald Trump supporters, having seen considerable evidence of irregularities in the election, could invalidate the past election. Then the presidential election would go to the House of Representatives of Congress, where according to the US Constitution, each state has one vote in choosing the president. Since most states will vote for Trump, he will be the next president of the United States. The question, therefore, was when it would be possible to file documents with the country's Supreme Court.

In Pennsylvania, it turned out that 165,000 Republicans sent their ballots in the mail, but their votes were not counted in the voting register, and the ballots themselves were lost.

Another person on Trump's team investigating possible election fraud told a live broadcast of one of the channels: the company was responsible for counting the votes in the US, with the company's office in Toronto, Canada, using the Dominion program and overseeing the election from servers in Germany.

The servers controlled elections in twenty-seven states.

Two Venezuelan citizens own this company. The Dominion program was created with Chinese money to manipulate Venezuela and secure Hugo Chávez in early 2000. The same program was used in Argentina. The Dominion program's people are associated with the Soros Foundation and the Global Initiative—the Clinton Foundation.

All the liberal media were broadcasting about Joe Biden's great victory. On social media, Trump supporters spoke about a detachment from a US military base in Germany that searched a local CIA office.

Trump's legal team has produced hundreds of documents that included affidavits (witnesses under oath), expert opinions, photos, and video evidence confirming numerous frauds during the 2020 presidential election. First of all, it's a power struggle. The struggle for the presidency in the United States was watched, without exaggeration, by the whole world.

Now it's decided not just who the president is taking a seat in the White House for the next four years but what the world will be like in the coming years and possibly in the foreseeable future.

Power makes it possible to get rich. Power makes it possible to become a successful dominant member in the community of the powerful. Power makes it possible to provide a fantastic future for their descendants. All three instincts inherent in the biological nature of *Homo sapiens* prompted Trump's opponents to act.

The United States has many friends worldwide and, of course, many enemies. Everyone waited for the results on which the fate of many peoples depended. The fraud in the November 3, 2020, general election in the United States was staggering. Hundreds of thousands, more than likely millions of popular votes, were fraudulently passed on to democratic candidate Joe Biden.

It has been more than 250 years since the founding

of the United States. Its ethnic composition has changed significantly. At the time of its founding, the country had fewer than four million people. In 2020, the population was more than 328 million people. Democratic policies include indulging the poor, handouts in social housing, and food stamps coupons (later replaced with credit cards, which do not demean the dignity of those living on benefits). Free medicine, free education, and many other benefits deprived recipients of the desire to seek a decent place in society. Benefits recipients were blamed on the government and the system, which did not allow them to show their talents and merits.

A massive army of such dependents hated republicans and saw democrats as their patrons. In their opinion, the rules of the Clintons' and Obama's presidencies only showed them that it was necessary to change the situation acceptably to bring power to the democrats.

On the side of the democrats were all likely minorities, loudly demanding rights for their romantic ideas of civil rights change, immigration, and climate-control policy—multiple ideological opponents advocated the change of the existing system and the creation of a socialist state.

For years, teachers in schools and college professors have taught young people that capitalism is an obsolete system and that socialism is a just society of the future. Media, newspapers, social liberal media, and giants of

Silicon Valley have promoted hatred of everything related to Trump. It came to the point that Facebook, Twitter, and Google blocked the pages of the country's president.

There was still hope that Congress would consider electoral fraud in swing states. According to the Constitution, the election results and voting would go to the House of Representatives, where the most votes, one from each state, would give an advantage to Donald Trump.

A joint meeting of the houses of Congress approving the election's results on November 3 was held on January 6, 2021. Under the Constitution, Vice President Pence presided over a joint meeting of both houses of Congress.

Given the sheer voter fraud, Trump supporters were confident that the vice president would not vote for the electoral votes' approval. There were voices of Trump supporters warning Mike Pence's "treason," but no one wanted to believe it.

Donald Trump addressed his supporters, urging them to gather for a peaceful demonstration in Washington on January 6 to demonstrate to members of Congress their attitude toward the elections.

It happened on January 6, when many Trump supporters gathered in Washington to express their opinions on the election.

At that time, both houses of Congress were sitting in the Capitol Building, approving the vote results from November 3.

A group of Trump supporters broke into the Capitol Building, provoked by BLM and Antifa fighters. They wore MAGA baseball caps depicting supporters of the president. To the surprise of the masses who burst into the Capitol, they did not meet any serious resistance. The FBI had information about the Capitol's impending invasion but took no measures to protect the people's representatives for some reason.

In social networking, video footage has been preserved where one of the uniformed police officers pushes the fence aside and invites those who wish to go to the Capitol. All of this suggests that it was a trap. One of the attackers was shot dead while trying to enter through a window. Who shot her and why was not very clear.

Members of Congress were evacuated to a safe shelter. A small group of infiltrators in the building wandered along the Capitol. Without an apparent leader, they did not know what else to do. The police and guards expelled the uninvited guests, and the people's deputies returned to their workplaces. Joe Biden was named president-elect, with Kamala Harris as vice president. They were very excited and outraged at President Trump, who should be justly punished for his supporters. Of course, all disputes about election fraud were inappropriate in such a situation.

Nancy Pelosi, the Speaker of the House of Representatives, insisted on declaring a "second attempt" to impeach the perpetrator of such an unheard-of attempt on the country's power. *President Donald Trump is guilty of inciting many of his supporters.*

The presidency of the new administration was confirmed. The inauguration of the new administration of Joe Biden and Kamala Harris occurred on January 20, 2021. Donald Trump's administration left the White House, making room for new hosts for the next four years.

Since the election, Trump and his supporters have made little attempt to overturn the rigged vote results, using the courts to prove the deception. Supporters of the president exchanged views animatedly on social media, discussing all sorts of scenarios and actions on the trail, up to the announcement of the country's situation, with the introduction of army units in cities where riots might occur.

The president's lawyers still tried challenging the election results, but it did not matter.

The courts, the political elite, the heads of law-enforcement agencies, the media, and social networks were ardent opponents of President Trump. The high court may have been intimidated or feared for their loved ones' lives; others were probably merely corrupt.

The day before the new administration's inauguration, Donald Trump and his family left the White

House, refusing to participate in the inauguration ceremony and leaving a letter to the new president.

Joe, you know I won.

Donald Trump came into the world of politics from the world of business. Trump attributed his rise to politics to failing to tolerate the Clinton-Obama policies that were destroying the economy and supporting dictatorial regimes in other countries to the detriment of the United States. During Trump's administration, the economy dramatically increased, GDP performed impressively, and the unemployment rate fell by 3.7 percent. Dependence on imports diminished, living standards rose, and the army strengthened. Unlike all American presidents before him, he fulfilled almost all his campaign promises. He proposed a logical slogan for business, America First, or Make America Great Again—MAGA. The slogan has been consistently followed and won many supporters among his country's population, with more than seventy-five million of his ardent supporters.

Donald Trump promised to drain the Washington swamp. This so-called Deep State is a club of elected people finally formed during the Clinton-Obama administration. They led the bureaucracy to the army, intelligence, finance, and legal system. Donald Trump has never been a member of this organization, and he threatened to drain the swamp, which made him numerous enemies. Since its founding by Democrat Jimmy Carter, the Deep State, has met the challenges of creating a democratic government. There has been a tumultuous rush toward the re-education of young people in schools, colleges, and universities.

Teachers and professors have taught young people that capitalism is bad and socialism is suitable for many years.

All media were involved for the same purpose: liberal media, TV, newspapers, and Silicon Valley giants. Acting at the same time, they brainwashed the youth, which led to society's moral degradation.

Traditional American values: independence, freedom, the pursuit of success, law-abiding, morality, and religious tolerance, replaced and promoted socialist slogans, where the American way of life became immoral.

America has changed along with its ethnic composition. On November 3, 2020, during the US general election, thousands, if not millions, of votes were rigged and handed over to the democratic nominee. At the same time, there was some slight hope that Congress would consider election fraud in some states and not approve it. And results would be to elect a president by so-called state vote, but it became clear from the outset that even many republicans would not mind getting rid of Trump.

A coup d'état took place.

MELTING POT

The idea of a melting pot arose due to the merger of different languages, cultures, peoples, nations, races, traditions, creeds, and many waves of immigrants from all over the world. English, in its American version, helped immigrants assimilate into the country. Introduced later, Spanish as the country's second language helped numerous Hispanic citizens blend into the multicolored carpet of the US population. Various groups have preserved their historical homeland traditions in real life and sought to settle in their districts, communicate, and buy food in *"their"* stores, the traditional products. They support their national holidays, culture, and symbols. Today we know that the idea of a melting pot has not stood the test of time.

American society supported the idea of ethnic, national identity, any group preserving the traditions of the ethnic group, their nation. It was laid by the Founding Fathers when the country was created. Preserved culture, religion, and customs of ethnic groups created a colorful palette, uniting peoples under one country's flag, the United States. Unfortunately, the collapse of the United States is inevitable.

In shackles brought forcibly to this country, the Black population will never term with second-class citizens' former position. No favors and reparations will lead to peace and harmony.

Preferential quotas for employment in government agencies and educational institutions are mandatory today in any field of culture, science, and sports, but this only increases racism, xenophobia, and hostility. The country's white population is already experiencing all the negative aspects of a wrong attitude toward themselves. There is no solution to this problem. In addition to this problem, there are many other problems with different minorities: political, gender, race, sexual, ethnic, religion, age, culture, and others. All minorities also demand preferential quotas in social society.

Such a transformation will predictably lead to many states' secession and forming a new Confederation of Free States. The two countries are unlikely to reach a peace agreement with their army and opposing ideologies. Splitting up into different entities will create intractable problems. The very idea of the country's disintegration will cause rejection, and a possible confrontation will lead to a civil war.

The consequences will be catastrophic. The reconcilability of ideologies excludes the possibility of a peace agreement and mutual concessions. The party that can convince the army and commands to side with them will inevitably have to use dictatorship and subordination to establish order and stability.

At the moment, the country is divided into two almost irreconcilable halves. No one will want to give in and accept the rules of building a society on principles acceptable only to one of the parties. Coercion and dictatorship will inevitably lead to armed confrontation. At the same time, none of the warring parties will peacefully resolve the contradictions with the other half of the population.

The biological nature of the *Homo sapiens* species ideally corresponds with the capitalist ideology and system. Socialistic ideology, in the absence of free enterprise, freedom of speech, and freedom of assembly, leads to the tyranny of the oligarchy, state dictatorship, and violence against the impoverished population. All its advantages, democratic freedoms, change of power, and equal opportunities for all population segments cannot do without the hard work of numerous unlucky members of society, forced to serve those, who are powerful. The strongest survive; it gives them the right to decide and choose the path. Those who cease to struggle for existence or the weak accept their fate or die out.

The United States of 2021 is a divided country. One side claims there was no fraud in the election. The other side says there has been massive fraud. Both sides cannot be correct. Do we know the truth?

Only the future will be able to prove who is right. In the modern world, there is no balance. European countries are not the benchmark for the balance between rich and poor. The waves of migrants from Asia and Africa that have swept the European continent threaten to sink the Old World's overloaded ship.

The *Homo sapiens* of all millennia existed according to the laws of their kind. Dominants have always been in the lead, and subordinates followed. Dominant: governing, dominating, commanding, contracting, ruling, driving, and many other synonyms exist in any language, and many antonyms—subjugation and obedience are great examples.

The republican form of government, accidentally found on a newly discovered and affluent continent, has created an illusion of a society of equal opportunity. It could be accurate, but not everyone can meet such demands.

The American dream of universal equality and happiness lasted almost a quarter of a millennium. Unfortunately, this dream is coming to an end.

Another illusion of *Homo sapiens* crashed. Inequality is inherent in the biological nature of the human brain. Karl Marx believed that every person's brain is structured the same. He believed scientists could develop a new breed of people capable of creating an ideal communist society of equal opportunities. He was wrong. American democracy has demonstrated, during its existence, the advantages of the free market system of capitalism.

Established forms of governance and political freedoms for entrepreneurship have created conditions for establishing a fair and controlled government. This state has kept the balance in society.

Biological instincts: Food, reproduction, and domination manifest in all the turbulent moments *Homo sapiens* pass. *Homo sapiens* fulfill its biological purpose. The political elite, concentrated power structures, used position to perform instinctive tasks inherent in our species' limbic system. Control over the food supply means life or death. Reproduction is necessary (descendants are opportunities to increase capital), and dominance (it's the struggle for a higher place in the hierarchy to increase capital). In recent history, this system has existed long enough, but the twenty-first-century events showed the deceptiveness of this system's seeming well-being and resilience.

The natural biological selection that turned the ape into a reasonable, humane being left us an inheritance in the form of the brain's limbic system.

Today, the rights of those who cannot or do not want to be a community member, imposing their views of society's behavior, are declared the most important and obligatory to be executed.

Today, being white could be challenging. Not having a fashionable sexual orientation is shameful; being rich is merely unacceptable. Flirting is "harassing" (insulting), displaying anger, destroying someone else's property—freedom of expression. This series can be continued indefinitely.

Liberalism has a double interpretation. There are democratic freedoms, rights, parliamentary rights, and equality for all before the law.

There is another meaning: pointless tolerance, harmful connivance, excessive liberality, and permissible deviation (from the norm). Today's liberalism is another interpretation of behavior in society. Ideas of social equality have always roamed our species' troubled heads. In the willingness to remake rules, from time to time, the leaders called on the people to revolutionize the world, overthrow the existing unjust system, and create a society of equal opportunities. The logic of revolutionary societal transformations is demand and offer to distribute goods, resources, and opportunities.

It quickly became apparent that such transformations require rugged protection from those who did not voluntarily part with the unjustly acquired and inherited values.

The confrontation of opposite opinions inevitably led to an armed conflict with all the ensuing under such an outcome. As we know from the history of the revolution, *if the enemy does not give up, it must be destroyed.* Civil wars and revolutions were always the bloodiest and most brutal. Children rose against their parents, brother versus brother.

The governments used their regimes with a force that created countless victims. The November 3, 2020, events seemed like a typical presidential election every four years. But there has been a change in the political regime. The Democratic Party, which has long shifted to the extreme left radical political position, has decided to remove the interfering president and finally implement the idea of universal equality and prosperity. First, it allows taking total control over all government branches in the country to make radical changes and lead the world toward liberalism and the unchecked rule of all living on this earth. This task was comparable to humanity's most outstanding achievements. The US could expect violent upheaval for the foreseeable future.

There is already pressure against the seventy-five million who voted for Donald Trump. The Democratic Party will push through laws restricting rights, freedoms, and the possibility of speaking and opposing views. Nancy Pelosi, the Speaker of the House of Representatives, called them "internal terrorists."

The House of Representatives voted to impeach

President Trump again, accusing him of "inciting sedition." The Senate must deliver its verdict on the fault of the country's president.

On January 20, 2021, Donald Trump left the White House, where new president Joe Biden moved in. Donald Trump became the first US president investigated for impeachment twice and could become the first president to be impeached and convicted after finishing his presidency. The Senate's decision has been postponed to the first days of February 2021. Democrats seek an indictment because it means Trump's de facto ban on holding public office for life.

In today's unstable world, proponents of the capitalist ideology of building a society call for faith in God, family values, equal rights and opportunities for all, the self-regulating power of the free market, and the value of human life. Capitalism is the last and unique historical development stage of *Homo sapiens*, really objective, identifying with civilization and culture.

Democratic liberal parties profess a socialist political ideology of building a society whose ultimate goal is fair social and economic equality—creating a classless just society.

It's replacing market forms of economic management with the public (read: state) control over production and equitable resource allocation.

The species *Homo sapiens* has already passed through this stage in its history. Recall the Great

French Revolution of 1792, the Russian Revolution of 2017, Venezuela's democratic socialism by Hugo Chavez in 2002, North Korea's Kim Il-sung and his descendants, China's Mao Zedong, Vietnam's Ho Chi Minh, Democratic Kampuchea (Cambodia), Pol Pot, leader of the Khmer Rouge.

They all pursued a policy of destruction of rights and freedoms and terror against their people.

Today's liberalism is another interpretation of behavior in society. You have already read about it in the second book of this trilogy, but it is good to repeat some of what you read, maybe some who never read, and perceive the connection with current events. Our species, *Homo sapiens*, began victorious conquest on this planet when the only weapon available to them was a large 1,650 cubic centimeters brain. *Homo sapiens* didn't come into this world with a brain that large. Our species has been going through development for millions of years.

The transformation of a small four-legged animal, proconsul, with a brain of three hundred cubic centimeters trying to survive. Among predators and other similar animals capable of dining on its flesh required brain improvement for survival in a harsh environment. The proconsuls existed in unimaginably distant times, twenty million years ago. The wool warmed them in East Africa, where apes' ancestors only had teeth and paws for survival protection. They had no advantage over other wildlife inhabitants except for a brain that evolved and grew in volume for millennia as the proconsul tried to survive. Just the instinct of self-preservation pushed his brain to search for immediate solutions to survival. The inherent biological instincts push living creatures to develop a necessary quality among similar species in the struggle for food, a female for procreation, and the manifestation of dominance (superiority), a necessary quality among this species' individuals. Biological nature encourages the brain's development, resists failure in a given environment, helps to avoid mistakes, and generates clues for more intelligent behavioral instincts in various circumstances.

Millennia passed, and the brains of great apes grew, accumulated much information, and put the brains' owners in the first rows of the food chain. They defended against cruel and strong opponents equipped with fangs, claws, horns, shells, poisonous teeth, and other attributes. It can be assumed that the most dangerous humanoid opponent could be another humanoid species, also considering such a biological creature as an object for nutrition. Cannibalism accompanied the history of humanoids of all ages; in some places, it has survived in our day. The planet's climate has changed and pushed our species and other wildlife to search for new habitats where conditions exist for survival. Scientists—archaeologists, paleoanthropologists, and paleogeneticists generalize the theory of human origin, relying on new finds, pushing further and pushing back datings and exit sites from Africa of *Homo sapiens* and other hominids. But one thing we know today.

The brain of Neanderthals and the brain of *Homo sapiens* were equal in volume to 1,650 cubic centimeters. Although not yet burdened with modern knowledge, large brains enable survival in changing conditions.

The surviving species of *Homo sapiens* lived in large populations of hunter-gatherers, moving further afield on the planet.

They lived in large populations, using fire, processing food, making stone and bone tools, hunting together, communicating, and adapting to local climatic conditions. Joint hunting and food sharing among members of the population contributed to the transformation of *Homo sapiens* into people living in primitive communal settings, communicating first by sounds and then words.

As in any animal community, some dominant individuals sought to subjugate other community members. Violators were expelled or eaten during an everyday meal. Life outside of the population was impossible. This fact contributed to the emergence of speech and the first religions; totem religions and established taboos kept the population in submission and obedience.

A lone man could not survive in the wild with many different predators. In subordination to the early forms of rules, the leadership's dominance suppressed the brain's initiative and the need to fight. This subordination could not pass without a trace for the human population. The brain of a modern person has decreased by 50 to 250 cubic centimeters. Fortunately, the structure of the brain is not inherited. Every brain is different. At birth, a person appears with a ready-made structure of the brain, formed in the womb.

The human brain's development, fate, and entire life depend on parents' genes and the environment. Our species has gone through five thousand years of building a civilizational society, from enslaved people for labor to universal equality. We have reached a population of eight billion people on the planet. We have achieved production of the mass destruction of our species —nuclear, bacteriological, chemical, laser, and cosmic. Our tomorrow is unknown because our species is divided politically, socially, psychologically, demographically, economically, ethnically, religiously, racially, nationally, along gender lines, and by culture and education.

Maybe we can find a way for everyone on Earth to live happily and peacefully.

The basis of human behavior has always been and always will be the economy of instinctive motives laid in us by nature—food, reproduction, dominance.

NEW TIME

Centuries and millennia have passed. *Homo sapiens* have long forgotten about their early past and, with the help of religion, considered themselves being created in the image and likeness of God himself.

In this scenario, people are not part of the planet's animal world but are the masters of everything that exists, created according to God's command. Any religion teaches it; it is written in all religious textbooks taught by the dominant religious teachers. Although the brain of *Homo sapiens* has decreased over time, science and knowledge over five millennia of civilizations have made the human brain incredibly sophisticated and inventive. The amount of knowledge that allowed man to invent computers was almost equal to the brain. We needed to understand the essence of DNA structure and the elementary unit of all living organisms' structure—a living cell. Civilization has brought humanity previously unthinkable benefits and advantages. Flying into space, swimming under the ice, making tunnels in the mountains, and the possibility of blocking rivers. Man became like God.

The limbic system obtained from our hominid ancestors required human actions related to all living organisms' biological natures. This required food (energy), reproduction (in the absence of offspring, the species dies out), and domination (getting advantages among its species). These three basic laws have always been in charge and will be in charge of the species of *Homo sapiens*, as such is the biological nature of man.

Modern man greatly differs from his ancestors, who lived thousands of years ago. Humanity has tried to create a reasonable formula for peace and universal prosperity, having gone through the bloody path of destroying their kind, cities, countries, and civilizations. Dictatorship led to democracy and gave way to absolutism, which was swept away by the republic. Then the rule of the dynasty's reign was replaced by the socialist dictatorship of the proletariat, which gradually turned into tyranny.

The search for a system capable of bringing common good and prosperity more likely accidentally happened to the first settlers of the newly discovered continent, America.

People who sought religious freedoms found freedom of opportunity and defended their rights in the war for independence from monarchical rule and the right to build a society on the principles of equality. The right of free enterprise and the right to preserve and accumulate the wealth earned have created the basis for that country's prosperity.

The brain of *Homo sapiens*, according to the instincts inherent in the limbic system, is arranged that way to take care of offspring and forces parents to transfer everything to children.

The capitalist philosophy of the economic system is based on private property and the freedom of entrepreneurship—the desire of any individual to increase capital and profit, transferable to their descendants. Hence, their life should be better than the ones they lived themselves. Children would receive a better education, could take advantage of the property acquired by their parents, and become respected people in society. The country provided all these opportunities.

Followers of Karl Marx, as faithful adepts, implemented his ideas to lead the collapse of society in any country that gave up the natural biological nature of *Homo sapiens*. The ideological and mythological value system imposed by Marxists does not work. No one wants to create values and then give them to those who only want to collect.

The common sense and instinct of *Homo sapiens* want to leave everything for their family and descendants. Houses, any created material values, go to inherit by their family. Socialists of all stripes declare liberalism starts from the concept of the general welfare. Behind this is a simple and primitive solution.

A large portion must be taken from those who have a lot, then divided among those who don't. This easy-to-like solution has one crucial drawback. Someone has to create value over and over again to share something. No one will create anything, knowing it will be taken away and distributed to others. Birds carry food in their beak to their offspring, which only squeaks, revealing the beak. Parental instinct makes parents care for their offspring, not someone else's. Today we also know many cases of adoption and foster parenting by godparents and orphanages. But it doesn't change the basic instinct of living organisms, especially humans.

It is the biological nature of *Homo sapiens*. Karl Marx or Lenin can not change the biological nature of humans. All Marxist experiments create a welfare society, then the state becomes a dictator, caring about society, ending in bloody tyranny, persecuting dissenters, and lacking freedoms. Recently, voices have been heard among far-left neo-democrats and globalists calling for the rending of private property. It is not a new idea of the communists, who have already tried to build a society on a new principle. A family, a relic of the past, children are kept in social institutions, and living in social housing does not distract from the primary task of building a happy future for humankind. *From each according to his ability to each according to his needs.*

The Chinese population came closest to this bright image of a happy human life in the twenty-first century.

Encouraged by the chanting slogans praising the Chinese Communist Party, the population dressed in uniforms stepped to the sound of a military orchestra and saluted their native party and beloved leader.

Unlike China, the USSR could never implement this fantastic idea, although the world proletariat leader, comrade Josef Stalin, tried to mow down almost half of the country's population. The cumbersome state machine, distributing and rationing everything and everyone, tried to cover all spheres of the country's life, which invariably led to the population's impoverishment, the lack of necessary goods and services, a decrease in the standard of living, and a reduction in its duration.

The massive management apparatus allowed many officials and managers to create unprecedented corruption opportunities, which were not used only by the lazy. The man in the corruption system realized opportunities were given to share with those he owed his position and nomination. Suppression apparatus—special forces, corrupt courts, and torture prisons—created an atmosphere of fear and obedience. Lies, hypocrisy, adaptability, and meanness dictated behavioral motives, where everyone could be a checker and a whistleblower. The mutual responsibility of the whole society created odious human types, where hypocrisy was a virtue and the desire to prove the truth ridiculous, stupid, and dangerous to others.

Specially trained and equipped troops were created to suppress dissenters in case of unrest or demonstrations. Corrupt courts handed down harsh sentences for publications, speeches, or other actions undesirable to the authorities.

It is the fate of any socialist system created in defiance of the natural laws of *Homo sapiens'* development. Why, time and time again, do people seek to create such a society? The answer, as always, lies in the instinct inherent in the human brain's limbic system: food, reproduction, and dominance. In creating any movement, its leaders deliberately strive for power. People respond to all the desires that guide such leaders. It is the motive, but countless false and unrealizable promises surround it. The ability to promise generously is the necessary quality of any leader.

It is human nature to believe in a bright future of equal opportunities. Leaders say to people: "*Look how much capital this individual has amassed. Why would he need that? You're the one who made him so wealthy. He robbed you and your family. Let's take it away from him, say 95 percent, and give it to everyone who needs it. That's only fair.*" Marx's faithful disciples relied on the proletariat.

Contrary to peasants, who had a piece of land to plow where the whole family could even have their cattle, the proletarians had nothing. They were the perfect environment for Marxists. In today's society, many individuals are not adapted to survive in a competitive environment. This simple philosophy finds fertile ground among the poor, unlucky, weak-willed, dependent, and often lazy. Illegal immigration world-wide pushes people in poor, corrupt countries to seek a better share for themselves and their offspring. They flee civil wars, devastation, lawlessness, corruption, and famine. In North America, illegal immigrants in 2019 increased dramatically. In Europe, the uncontrolled movement of migrants from Asia and Africa contributed to chaos and casualties.

Uncontrollable waves from the Middle East and Africa are sweeping the European Union. The EU authorities, trying to regulate and distribute the flows of migrants between the EU member states, faced stiff resistance from the union's new members. Internal borders were restored with border control.

The history of the United States is very different from the history of development in other countries. The beginnings of that country are very similar to those of other colonial countries. But this country was inhabited by entirely different people. The spirit of freedom and independence, the desire for entrepre-neurship, the desire to break through, hard work, and healthy adventurism created a new nation, different from the submissive in many generations of European nations.

America is a land of opportunities open to anyone. All it takes is a desire to succeed, get rich, become financially independent, and create a good family.

Naturally, not everyone succeeds. Everyone inherited a specific and, most importantly, individual brain structure. Someone was lucky and been helped to develop and find themself in this life. For another, fate did not prepare loving and caring parents. People are trying hard to make their way, and they are more prepared for life than those who work under the strict command of someone or are being helped and nourished. Of course, many could give up after an unsuccessful struggle for a place under the sun.

Unfortunately, people will make a mistake without understanding it, eventually destroying this admirable and exemplary value system. Many of the Founding Fathers were enslavers and could not have imagined that such a human relationship system was exploited and violated fundamental human rights when one person was another person's property. They wrote the Declaration of Independence on July 4, 1776, which said *that all people are created equal. They are all endowed with the Creator's inalienable rights, including life, freedom, and the pursuit of happiness.*

The Founding Fathers were pioneers in creating the constitution of equality and could not foresee how public relations would change in the foreseeable future. Could they have foreseen what slavery would lead to in the country they were creating? This assumption is unlikely. How could this happen? Almost a quarter of a millennium has passed. Slavery was the norm in the minds of people of that time.

Slavery has existed in the history of *Homo sapiens* since prehistoric times. Prisoners and debtors were turned into enslaved people and later forced people to work for their masters. In the United States, enslaved Black people from Africa were brought in by enslaved–people traders and sold on markets. The southern states used bonded enslaved–people labor in agriculture and household services.

The price of this tragic mistake sooner or later led to the most profound chasm in the country's society. The Founding Fathers laid down what was happening in America. For thousands of years, enslaved–people's labor was common in European and Muslim countries. As enslaved-people owners, they decided to put the solution to slavery aside for twenty years for the next generation. They created the US Constitution, and the price for this mistake will be paid by the generation living in the country today.

In Tsarist Russia, serfs were enslaved people who were bought and sold. Tsar Alexander II made a decree abolishing serfdom on March 3, 1861.

Slavery and most countries' colonial policies undoubtedly influenced the world's future. The consequences of this phenomenon have yet to be assessed and rethought. Any sane modern person regrets and condemns what happened in the past. But as you know, history has no subjunctive inclination. Or, as the English say, *"What's the use of crying over spilled milk?"* The United States' Black population grew up with the consciousness that they were descendants of enslaved people brought forcibly in shackles and sold to masters for enslaved–people's labor.

The American Civil War of 1861—1865 between the North and South freed the Black population from slavery. But segregation remained, separating the country's white people and Blacks.

There have been numerous efforts to help the country's new citizens, who are Black, fit into the US population's general culture.

That took many centuries, and many successive generations tried to solve it with handouts and advantages. The countless Black citizens of the country have achieved incredible success in various fields: arts, music, sports, politics, healthcare, education, goods manufacturing, services, government, and political positions.

But all this did not improve the overall situation. Today, the US is home to about 330 million people, with a Black population of 12.7 percent. The first Black president, Barack Obama, became president of the United States and a Nobel laureate.

By 2020, the country's African American population was an impressive forty-two million. Many Black society members still face social problems related to low levels of education, high crime, and family crises.

The stratification in society could cause a protest movement. Mass protests against racism and far-fetched police brutality in 2020 have fueled the emergence of a mass movement for Black people's rights, *Antifa, Black Lives Matter,* and many other small groups.

For the Democratic Party, these Black rights groups have proven ideal for creating strike groups in the struggle for supremacy in all bodies of power: the presidency and both houses of Congress.

Antifa and Black Lives Matter organizations have received massive support from their patrons in the past few years, organizing attacks on businesses, civilians, and police, destroying everything in their path, smashing private property, and setting fire to police cars and plots. Vast sums of money were transferred to the accounts of these organizations. The police and authorities on the ground were forbidden to prevent the people's free and peaceful protest and expression of will.

They left behind smashed windows, looted shops, burned police cars, and destroyed houses, terrorizing the residents. The BLM movement has existed for seven years, holding various street rallies and demonstrations and outlining their ideas in social network publications. In June 2020, BLM staged protests in the US and Britain over the Black man George Floyd's death. The Minneapolis Police detained him in Minnesota. During the arrest, he showed fierce resistance. The police took harsh measures upon arrest.

Floyd was taken to the hospital, where he later died. Although the investigation found that death resulted from various diseases and intoxication, the death led to numerous protests.

More than twenty million Americans participated in these protests in the United States. According to the polls, 50 percent of Americans supported the BLM movement.

No one was embarrassed that the police detained the rioters' hero, George Floyd, born in 1973, with a tall and athletic physique. He was arrested several times for theft and possession of drugs. In 2007, he was charged with armed robbery and sentenced to five years in prison. He was a recidivist criminal, tormentor, rapist of women, drug addicted, drug dealer, violent and vicious. After a call from a store worker who accused Floyd of paying for the purchase with a fake bill, police arrested him. When Floyd was arrested, he resisted, and the police had to use force. The police were accused of abuse of power.

The death of George Floyd served as a trigger for spontaneous expressions of anger. There were gangs, arson of cars, attacks on police, unprovoked violence, and murder on the streets of cities. Gangs smashed shop windows with the obligatory looting of goods inside them. This bacchanalia was accompanied by demands to deprive police of funds and the white population's widespread repentance for hundreds of years of Black's slavery. They demand mandatory reparations and benefits for Black people, including resettling African Americans in white-owned homes. The white population is obliged to recognize committed crimes, kneel and kiss African Americans' feet or shoes. Many TV stations show such scenes on American streets.

The youth gangs beat those who refused to perform such rituals. They also seized parts of cities run by the democrats, turning them into *zones free of police presence.* In these ghettos, there was arbitrariness, violence, robberies, shootings between gangs, and murders.

Since George Floyd's death on May 25, 2020, unrest has not subsided, but heads of democratic-led states have refused any military assistance offered by President Trump to bring order. Police were not allowed to intervene; if someone was arrested for violent crimes, there were always means of bail. The courts release the bandits without understanding the crime.

There were loud opinions that such acts were carried out as revenge for centuries of slavery and humiliation. Robberies of expensive shops and fashion boutiques were justified because the outcasts never had a chance to buy such expensive things. The authorities called these pogroms peaceful protests of the citizens of the country.

"Rob the robbers" was the motto of the Bolsheviks, who destroyed the Russian tsarist empire in 1917.

This turning point year in US history, with the pandemic caused by the COVID-19 virus from China, has been accompanied by riots and looting, a bender of hostility, and threats on Donald Trump throughout his presidency. All influential and powerful groups perceived Donald Trump's unexpected appearance in the country's political arena as an evil New Year's joke. For them, he seemed like a clown and showman, not very smart and naturally not dangerous. Sounds like a conspiracy theory? What did the United States president do to the neo-Democratic Party that they hated him so much? During the sixteen years of the Clinton and Obama administrations, democrats had put the right and valuable people in all the key places. Perhaps, it's hard to explain where such organized and effective resistance to Trump's desire to be president for another four years suddenly appeared in 2020.

Donald Trump created many problems for democrats during his first term as president, depriving many of stable and abundant incomes. He broke many essential ties both at the domestic and international levels.

Imagining what he could do in his four years in office was frightening and could have ended badly for many influential people. Despite the president's investigation by Special Prosecutor Mueller, slander in the media, opposition to the House of Representatives, slander and deception in the country's security forces, attempts at impeachment, accusations of sexual harassment, threatening his family and children, he did not give up. He continued to fight for the country's economy, improving the Middle East and all parts of the world, fighting for honest relations between countries, peace, and returning the American soldiers home.

TRUMP AS A
HINDRANCE

Donald Trump was interfering with democrats in power structures, and they wanted to get rid of him. The global interests of many stakeholders and states have demanded radical solutions to the Donald Trump problem. Who are all these people, organizations, interests, ideologies, and states that Donald Trump opposed?

In the US, he represented the conservative capitalist economic development system ideology. Trump came from the business world, where everything is subject to increasing profits and decreasing the tax base to survive in the competition. Production and distribution are based on private property, law, and free enterprise. Regaining control of the House of Representatives in 2018, the democrat's top priority has been gaining control of the Senate and the White House. Such an advantage could allow the election in the future of a democratic president, obedient to the legislators' will. Such a task was the center stone in the ideology of democrats.

Homo sapiens have long been known as the species; getting power allows perform the three main functions laid down by human biological nature: food, reproduction, and dominance. The politician elite occupying the dominant position in society receives uncontrollable opportunities for sweet life (real estate, values, the cheerful and happy holiday of life) and the pinnacle of opportunities, providing offspring in the third and fourth generations.

Not only was Trump the main obstacle to this glorious dream, but he could also destroy the established status quo of elite political life. He threatened to "drain the Washington swamp," which meant dismissals from all the leading positions in the power and political structures of the right and essential people, tied in one strong knot. The principle of power-sharing and mutual assistance in distributing opportunities could collapse and bury all the hopes that seemed so accessible and feasible.

Trump's most dangerous thought was of changing terms in office for the legislative branches of government, limiting tenure in the Senate to two terms and the House of Representatives to three. In this way, he made enemies on all sides. People go into politics in the hope of achieving high positions. It could be compared to good business or a prestigious profession.

It is natural for *Homo sapiens* to follow the species' basic instincts (food, reproduction, dominance). Staying in power in today's world meets all these instincts—respect among others, secured existence, glorious old age, wonderful life for themselves and their descendants, financial opportunities without the risk of losing everything in an unfortunate case, and the achievement of desires.

According to the Constitution, the country's presidency is limited to two terms of four years. Being in either chamber of Congress, the number of terms is unlimited. John Dingell has served in Congress for more than fifty-five years. Joe Biden has been in Congress for forty-seven years, and that's not a record.

Donald Trump has bitten on the holy. He signed his sentence by proposing limiting the stay in Congress to two terms, depriving ex-members of the glorious pensions and the privileges they expected, and simply sending them back to their former job in the previous life.

Senator Ted Cruz picked up the baton, saying, "Today, my colleagues and I have re-amended the Constitution to impose term limits on members of Congress. The amendment would limit US senators to two six-year terms and US House of Representatives members to three two-year terms."

Given that the new constitutional amendment was introduced at the end of January 2021, when democrats, essentially, own both Congress and the White

House, such an amendment will not pass. For democrats, having just won all the dominant positions, Ted Cruz proposes to make them commit to professional hara-kiri. It's courageous and naive. There is no chance, but this position is voiced, and who knows, maybe someday there will be another brave person able to carry out this amendment. Ted Cruz may have to pay a heavy price for such a bold constitutional amendment.

Rejecting all the legal principles, justice, and common sense, violating the US Constitution, conspirators were obsessed with one idea, removing the legitimately elected US president, Donald Trump, from power. Against Donald Trump stood a united front of all the government branches: legislative, executive, and judicial. On the president's side remained a small group of republicans and seventy-five million Americans who voted for him.

Lies, betrayal, and rigging of the November 3 vote may have created a democratic handover of power to the winner of the race, Joe Biden.

Against Donald Trump, for the first time in the history of the United States, was a united front: all the country's intelligence services, all democrats and a significant portion of republicans, all social networks, and all liberal media, with a few exceptions: the banking sector, financial tycoons, insurance companies, and most White House staffers.

Army generals refused to enter the National Guard in the cities where the mob smashed private and government buildings in the spring of 2020.

The military-industrial complex earns money from the production of weapons. Trump did not involve the country in any war, but, on the contrary, returned American soldiers home.

Leaders of many countries, opponents of the United States: China, Russia, Iran, Venezuela, officials of some countries of Europe, and third-world countries have grouped against Donald Trump.

What did Donald Trump achieve in his four years in office?

He had a considerable impact on the country's economy.

He significantly reduced unemployment to record lows in US history, including Afro-Americans, Hispanics, Asians, and for women.

Trump pointed out to NATO countries that the EU bloc unfairly underpays its share instead of the stipulated 2 percent of GDP. Thereby Trump saved the US many millions of dollars.

He held direct talks with North Korean dictator Kim Jong-Un for the first time in history. He was nominated for the Nobel Peace Prize three times.

President Donald Trump has exposed deep state corruption, including the CIA, FBI, ANB, the court at all levels, and ruling parties. He restored the US Army, increasing the budget by over seven hundred billion dollars.

He accused China of causing and spreading the COVID-19 virus and concealing information about the possibility of spreading the virus, leading to a global pandemic. More than 120 countries support the requirement to investigate the coronavirus pandemic causes and sue China. Compensation for the effects of the pandemic could rise to $30 trillion.

The world owes President Donald Trump the speedy vaccine development in the shortest time in history. Trump mediated the conclusion and the Middle East agreement between the Arab countries of the Persian Gulf and Israel for the first time in seventy-one years of endless wars and confrontations. Donald Trump waived the US president's $400,000-a-year salary.

"My father lost a fortune when he ran as the president of the United States. But he doesn't care."

— DONALD TRUMP JR.

Donald Trump has fulfilled practically all his campaign promises. The importance of President Trump's positive changes over four years cannot be overstated. During the sixteen years of the Clintons and Barack Obama, the democrats could dramatically change domestic politics.

President Trump was accused of racism, xenophobia (dislike of strangers and foreigners), homophobia (dislike of people with non-standard sexual preferences), sexism (gender discrimination), and far-right political views.

He is accused of promoting intolerance and antagonism to anything that did not fit Trump's vision of society's structure in the United States. He is the leader of those who do not share the principles of the left democrats; they are, in Madame Clinton's words: *deplorable people* (nasty, shameful, hateful, disgusting).

Hated by the democrats, forty-fifth US president Donald Trump has become the leader of freedom, prosperity, and peace for seventy-five million Americans and many sane people worldwide.

Jimmy Carter, a democratic president of the country, on September 19, 1979, signed an executive order establishing the SES Senior Executive Service, the Senior Leadership Service. The department hosted the best, most talented, and naturally divisive views of democratic leaders.

Of course, the pay scale for such an elite exceeded the average wage level for civil servants. These people had to stand at the head of all federal services to optimize these services' management. The elite SES community members have taken positions in most government departments and ministries. This powerful corporation is the deep state's backbone, leading the resistance and torpedoing Trump's attempts to stay in the White House for another term.

Barack Obama reorganized all government agencies, placing the right people in critical government positions, including intelligence services and the army. That was how the deep state, the army of top government officials loyal to the Democratic Party, was created. Barack Obama, before his departure, aware of the danger to his legacy and possibly the investigation into the various circumstances of his rule, held a meeting of the country's most significant leaders. Attending: Vice President Joe Biden, FBI Chief Jim Comey, CIA Director John Brennan, Secretary of State John Kerry, and National Security Adviser Susan Rice.

After this meeting, John Brennan noted: "Any evidence of cooperation between Trump's headquarters and Russia."

The meeting was the starting point for "Plan B" if Donald Trump was elected.

Then it was decided to start spying on Trump's family, headquarters, and associates. Obama warned: everything must be by the book.

After Donald Trump's apparent threat to drain the Washington swamp, the deep state power has fallen on him. Special Prosecutor Mueller's two-year investigation required constant answers and took a lot of force and time.

Engaged liberal media daily poured a sea of dirt, gossip, speculation, and outright lies on the incumbent president. Only one news channel, Fox News, has maintained the president's image by interviewing and showing Trump's presidency facts. Democrats and the media mocked and ridiculed everything Trump did, trying in every possible way to prevent him from carrying out important and necessary changes in many legislative, political, and economic areas of the country. On a par with Abraham Lincoln, the economic and political merits of Donald Trump could have given anyone in his place the glory of America's greatest president.

Social networks and internet platforms in recent years have grown into giant corporations, competed on a par with the media, and more often defeated mass media in the struggle for information and distribution of advertising. Visitors to social networks become loyal supporters of the ideas promoted by the networks. In a relatively short time, social media corporation owners became billionaires who didn't just want to maintain the network's image and revenues; they wanted to influence politics, dictate the terms of use of their networks, and not be responsible for content.

Modern society prefers communication on social networks such as Facebook, Twitter, Google, Vkontakte, Telegram, etc. Most of them overwhelmingly support the Democratic Party.

Trump signed an executive order *against censorship* on social media. He also demanded to exclude Article 230 from the law "on ethics in the field of communications." Social networks implicated in censorship or political action will not be protected from liability.

Mitch McConnell, the Senate majority leader, won enough votes with democrats to override the president's veto.

Trump's lawyers have gathered enough evidence of interference in the 2020 presidential election by China, Russia, Iran, and others. It allowed the president to take advantage of the decree of the state of emergency imposed by the country or specific areas to protect against external or domestic threats and maintain public order and national security.

The president's decree on the imposition of a state of emergency 13848 was signed by President Trump in September 2018 and was extended. The decree allowed the president to receive such information: "shall conduct an assessment indicating that a foreign government, or any person acting as an agent of or on behalf of a foreign government, has acted with the intent or purpose of interfering in that election...."

"Secretary of the Treasury, in consultation with Attorney General, Secretary of State, is authorized to submit the recurring and final reports to the Congress on the national emergency declared in this order."

In simple language, the last election's result indicates intervention.

It could be determined as canceled until authorities cleared the issue.

President Trump did not concede his election defeat but chose not to impose an emergency regime.

President-elect Joe Biden was sworn in on January 20, 2021.

What is happening in the country after Trump's departure? It was possible to predict with certainty that sooner or later, the democrats would come to power. Simply because there will be more of them, and a democratic system of electing government bodies will give them the majority of votes. But then it will not be America, but Russia, Belarus, Venezuela, or any other dictatorial state. No American president would even dream of suppressing radical left movements by force. It requires a dictator who is not afraid of bloodshed.

Is it a solution where left-wing radicals rush to power and have all the levers to solve this problem?

In Russia, there were famous eternal questions: "What to do? Who is responsible?" (A. Herzen and N. Chernyshevsky.)

In the United States, the twenty-seventh amendment to the Constitution was adopted. There is probably only one way to save the country—to pass another —the Twenty-Eighth Amendment, although the chances of ever happening are minimal.

But there is a similar process to amend the US

Constitution. Representatives and senators can propose an amendment. If a two-thirds majority passes, the amendment goes to the states. Three-quarters of state legislatures must approve the amendment to make a constitutional change. Who knows which direction history will turn in the future, especially if the left is eventually defeated in an election?

So, what is this amendment that could save the country? All the troubles in the country stem from the fundamental defect of democracy—universal suffrage. It means that the mass unemployed population living on benefits and the support of the state will always vote for those who promise and give them new privileges and handouts. Like a snowball, this inevitably leads to steady population growth, which prefers life on benefits rather than fighting for a better life. It will continue until the country collapses into the economic abyss and suffers the fate of ancient Rome.

Democracy is toothless and helpless—the lack of democracy leads to tyranny.

Democracy leads to tyranny when the number of dependents and those who want to use the system for their benefit exceeds the critical mass. It is the case pushing today's country, the United States, into the abyss of socialism. Therefore, the Twenty-Eighth Amendment should limit voting rights to citizens who do not live on state benefits. In other words, only those who earn their living and pay taxes can elect the government. The age qualification giving the right to vote is limited from age thirty-five to seventy. The population not wanting to work and pay taxes should not determine the state's fate. Another mandatory change must concern the House of Representatives. The right to dispose of the country's financial resources and budgeting should pass to a particular ministry associated with the tax administration. The submitted budget and allocated funds are approved by Congress and signed by the president.

The House of Representatives controls the country's finances. The existing order is "corruption-capacious," creating the main instability problems in society.

Since the mid-twentieth century, young people have been brainwashed in schools and universities. Most university professors promote liberal values. Professors convince students of the advantages of socialism over capitalism.

Political correctness has become a prerequisite for higher education. African Americans are touted as white supremacy victims who have the right to express their righteous anger with destruction and arson. The white population has been obliged to atone for the sins of crimes committed since the first enslaved Black person in shackles appeared on American soil.

In the 1970s, America ultimately ended segregation. It even went further by giving African Americans the pre-eminent rights to apply for public office, university admissions, and many other privileges inaccessible to the nation's white population.

The Black community takes all these innovations for granted. The attention and reverence, kneeling, kissing shoes, labeling white people "racist," and calling for the American anthem to be abolished.

That is supported by many of the white population. Loudly chanting propaganda among socialist values are university professors, publicizing the public's position with approval.

Such movements called on young people to tear down monuments of white "racists," inviting everyone and directing Black robbers to riot, seizing entire city areas where unchecked power was established.

A computer revolution began in the 1980s, fundamentally changing the planet's life. Giants of new technologies
such as Apple, Microsoft, Google, Facebook, and Twitter have divided civilization's history into before and after.

The technological revolution has contributed to globalization's phenomenon, associated with the transfer of production to countries where living standards are much lower than in developed countries. Cheaper labor and lower environmental requirements for protecting working conditions have contributed to transferring production to third-world countries. The resulting goods can be sold in profitably insolvent countries with hard currency. China and other Asian countries produce products that are sold all over the world. For example, 95 percent of US antibiotics were produced in China. US manufacturing was shutting down, increasing unemployment. Tech giants seized the information market, agreeing on whether they acted and deciding what was allowed to be published and what was prohibited. Facebook, Google, and Twitter have blocked President Donald Trump's channels, claiming it is supported by election fraud *being used to incite violence.*

By the 2020 presidential election, the Democratic Party was preparing to seize power, realizing Donald Trump's presidency's real threat for the next four years. It is clear and presents a danger to the very existence of democrats in power—losses of all that was achieved during the Clinton and Obama years. A plan was developed based on voter manipulation. The Dominion Voting System supplied automatic vote-counting machines. That system was made for the dictator of Venezuela, Hugo Chavez. Dominion Voting Systems Corporation, sales of ownership, and software security for electronic voting. Machines for voting, tabulation, and security.

Scytl Secure Electronic Voting developed software for counting elections. One of the shareholders of the company is the husband of Nancy Pelosi. The company is a Spanish supplier of e-voting systems and technologies. All data passes through servers located in

Frankfurt am Main, Germany. Scytl was based in Barcelona, Spain. The company is headquartered in Toronto, Canada. When trying to determine the impact of these programs on counting votes in the 2020 US elections, the company filed for bankruptcy and safely disappeared.

Trump's lawyers discovered multimillion manipulations in the counting of votes. Dominion has vehemently denied any allegations of the transfer to Biden or the destruction of votes of Trump supporters. Courts of all levels have refused to accept any claims from Trump's lawyers. Democratic Party leaders created the plan and drafted it to win the 2020 election. It could all be under the leadership of Barack Obama. It was decided to use the BLM and Antifa strike groups to create a state that creates fear and uncertainty in society regarding the stability of the Trump regime. A candidate for the future president of the country was chosen. Democrats picked Joe Biden. Why precisely that one when the organizers knew about Biden's weakness as a candidate?

With his corrupt ties and his other vices, naturally, he was the more convenient because he was easy to manage and easy enough to replace. If Joe Biden failed, he could be blamed for all his sins.

Of the many democratic presidential candidates, Kamala Harris was the most suitable. But her candidacy would be challenging to hold on to at the ballot. The black-skinned, Asian-born politician who served as California's attorney general was a US senator who did not have a good voting chance for a presidential position. As it turned out, the main thing is not who votes but who counts. But promoting Kamala Harris as president could cause many questions and complications. Seventy-eight-year-old Joe Biden, who also suffers from obvious signs of ill health, could play the "Trojan horse" role and lead Kamala Harris as vice president. After retiring, Joe Biden will hand over the reins to his rightful successor, Kamala Harris.

The COVID-19 crisis, which emerged in late 2019, has helped democrats close the country to quarantine and transfer a considerable portion to mail votes, contributing to voter fraud and fake ballots. The voting was a well-planned and organized action by the Democratic Party.

The death of the Black repeat offender George Floyd was a good reason for racial demonstrations, smashed windows, arson, and other allowed bacchanalia of outrageous youngsters from BLM, Antifa, and other groups.

No one was interested when the autopsy revealed Floyd's death came from a drug overdose. The crowds were burning cars, demolishing monuments to famous personalities of the past, accusing the latter of racism, enslaving Blacks, and demanding reparation to Black people for all the years of slavery.

Floyd became a new American banner and

symbol, a recidivist, rapist, and drug addict buried in a golden coffin.

In recent years, the US has seen a significant change in the ethnic composition of the population. America has always been a land of immigrants. Economic growth stimulated the need to increase the number of workers. New technologies need specialists in the field of information and communication technologies. The country was flooded with legal immigrants from India, China, Russia, Pakistan, and many others. Through Mexican borders quickly came mass illegal immigrants, mostly poorly educated but honest and hardworking people. Together with them, many criminals and asocial groups penetrate the US, leading to a marginal, criminal life. Drug trafficking, extortion, banditry, prostitution, and human trafficking are the sphere of youth gangs' activity.

Today, the United States is a vast population living on government benefits that depend on those who pay taxes.

The dependents represent a powerful and easily manipulated electorate for the Democratic Party. These are its future electorate. It is easy to manipulate them by distributing all kinds of privileges and handouts: the right to residency, free education, free medicine, free food, free housing, the right to citizenship, and other privileges. Whichever party promotes the idea of handouts more—for that party, the dependent will vote. It's only natural and expected behavior. Most of them require changes related to the cultural and religious customs adopted in the countries of origin. Their voices are getting louder. They hold elective offices, using the rights granted in a democratic society. The children of these immigrants, born in the United States, are raised in families where the culture, traditions, and religions differ from modern American ones. Having come to power, they loudly demand changes. They are against US policy in the country and the world. They are against the Americans' right to have weapons. They are against police, prisons, and border guards. They want to seize power and destroy this country by shattering American society's pillars.

The United State's problem is that no country has so many centrifugal forces to destroy established societal relations. The "melting pot," something America was so proud of, is already overheated and can explode into debris.

It was initially a bad idea. To gather in one, even a very fertile place on our planet, people of different cultures, races, nationalities, degrees of development, religions, ideas, desires, and opportunities guaranteed the common good.

Such a glorious fairy-tale theory attracted all who believed in the tale of Santa Claus. In real life, there are differences, misunderstandings, and the usual human envy of the successes and fortunes of those who could succeed with their work, talent, or a not-quite-honest way to succeed. Every person in the country cannot be successful, healthy, wealthy, and happy.

As the world classic Leo Tolstoy said: "All happy families are similar to each other; each unhappy family is unhappy in its way."

It's a very colorful metaphor; in reality, we all go through certain life stages. Origin, habitat, biological data, luck, and many other components affect our life. The dream of equal opportunity is extraordinarily tempting.

People growing up in a ghetto, a dysfunctional family, a poor social environment, inherited health problems, and other unfavorable circumstances blame society for an unsettled destiny.

For many of us, the name is legion (a Bible quote).

Such people exist in any social system. They blame the country, society, and people in power and dream of changing the existing order. Undoubtedly, one day, the burning (hidden) fire overheats the cauldron, and the flames will tear out and burn everything around. The belief that passing through the *"crucible of equal opportunities"* would allow so different people gathered here to equalize and think the same as one person was naive, but as it turned out, it was also dangerous.

WINNERS ARE NOT BE JUDGED

On the contrary, the winners do judge. The democrats were the winners in that race. The power "About which Bolsheviks talked for so long, passed into the hands of the people" —almost according to Vladimir Lenin, made by democrats. Joe Biden, the new forty-sixth president of the United States, for the first week of his stay in the White House, set a new record, overshadowing all previous presidents. He signed forty presidential decrees, including The South Carolina XL Pipeline for freezing the permit for laying Keystone, a chain of oil pipelines from Canada across the country to the Gulf of Mexico, and multiple refineries. This decree took tens of thousands of skilled union workers out of jobs in the United States. The record signing of presidential decrees is connected with the cancellation of President Donald Trump's previous decisions, including withdrawal from WHO (World Health Organization) membership, the Paris Climate Agreement, the construction of walls on the border with Mexico, and the state of emergency on this border. He lifted the ban on entry from six countries' citizens, predominantly Muslim populations. With feverish haste, Joe Biden's administration is preparing numerous decrees to sign by the forty-sixth president as if he fears that he may not have time to turn the country into a second Venezuela. Judging what is happening in the country, not only Republicans but also many Democrats are beginning to realize such an administration can lead now.

Does Joe Biden realize what he's doing? Sometimes there are doubts about his sanity, especially when he asks others, *"What am I signing?"* It seems that the new president is needed to do all the dirty work of destroying the country; then he can be sent to rest, putting on him all the sins in case of problems. Who benefits from it, the destruction of the world leader, the destruction of the US economy, the fall of the dollar payment system, the destruction of military power, the involvement of world powers in a new round of military confrontations, the severe crisis and the collapse of the world order? Many conspiracy theories come to mind, but it all seems so pointless and illogical that it remains only to shrug our shoulders.

The US is moving in the direction of socialist transformations in the country. The ideology of socialism does not tolerate confrontation, opposing opinions, or discussions.

After winning, the winners become judges. Ideological opponents cannot express their opinions and should be expelled from public life. House Speaker Nancy Pelosi called former President Trump's supporters "terrorists from within," which aligns with the socialist leaders' best revolution traditions.

Newly appointed by Joe Biden, the head of the US Department of Defense, Lloyd Austin, the first African American in this post, announced the need to suspend the activities of the Department of Defense for sixty days to *"cleanse white extremists"* in the ranks of the *"defenders of American democracy."*

Homo sapiens had already gone through something similar in the USSR, when "white officers" were subjected to "cleansing," with further reprisals in the GULAG camps. It is not yet clear what will happen to the retired US officers. Figuring out the politically incorrect biography counts and dissatisfaction with the new administration of "rebels" should take sixty days to "cleanse."

The fate of the discharged to the reserve will be decided by the Pentagon, perhaps by more competent authorities. Social networks tightly control bloggers in the network, removing channels for the slightest hint of fraud in the presidential elections in 2020. Democrats are brutally pressing ideological opponents at all levels of society.

On February 7, 2021, an "amazing" article signed by Jeff Carlson appeared in *Time magazine*. It was an astonishing story about the "secret shadow campaign against Trump." "They didn't falsify the elections; they strengthened them."

Time magazine said:

The story is secret and strange in its insouciance. It can be compared to the Olympic Games when the winners talk about various tricks, frauds, bribery of court, and other innocent tricks and stunts. In 'decent company,' it is not customary to talk out loud, and even more so in the press to talk about not quite sporty behavior during competitions.

In "The Secret History of the Shadow Campaign That Saved the 2020 Election," *Time* magazine describes how the actions of numerous groups and communities were united by one task, winning the 2020 election. The article's author calls these groups and the communities a "conspiracy unfolding behind the scenes that have limited protests and coordinated resistance of the leaders," leading to an alliance between left-wing activists and businesses.

The Democratic Party's "fears for the security of democracy" in the country rallied together "Legislative power, giants of social networks, Deep State."

All aspects of elections and changes in voting

systems have been worked out, with changes to the state's voting laws. These people do

not hide but consider their merit to change the power in the country. They want everyone to know and remember it. Joe Biden's new administration, followed by House Speaker Nancy Pelosi, is concerned about the threats of terrorism at home. "One of the greatest threats we face in our homeland... is the threat of domestic terrorism".

It's like the fear of a defeated but yet-to-be-destroyed enemy, former president Donald Trump. Nancy Pelosi pushed the Trump issue through the House of Representatives to impeach him, accusing Donald Trump of inciting his supporters to sedition on January 6, 2021. He addressed his supporters to arrive in Washington on January 6, 2021, and walk in front of the Capitol building "peacefully, keeping order." Nancy Pelosi accused Donald Trump of inciting sedition. She and her democratic colleagues are well aware that, like the first one, impeachment will not occur in the Senate, as it requires two-thirds of senators to vote for it.

In the Senate, in favor, fifty-five votes for impeachment to forty-five against it. It appears that many republicans could yield pressure and vote to impeach the former president, but many will face elections in 2022, and punishment for treason could be very career damaging. So, what did the democrats need for this whole week-long show? The country is in a pandemic. The economy is on the verge of a severe crisis, unprecedented unemployment, a divided country, borders no longer holding back, could break, and create chaos. But the main thing today for democrats is to impeach the former president, Donald Trump, for violating the US Constitution. The same procedure of impeaching a president, or senior officials, who have committed gross violations of the law, does not apply to persons who do not hold these positions.

The Senate cannot declare a criminal penalty. The weight of this farce with impeachment is meaningless and unconstitutional. Perhaps Democrats hoped to get sixty-seven votes in the Senate and impeach Donald Trump. In this case, he would lose the right to protection, pension, and other privileges as a former president. However, most importantly, he will not be elected to any position in the future. That was probably the main reason that prompted democrats to take this step. Whether it is just an emotional hatred of the defeated enemy behind it or even more insidious plans for revenge will show in the future.

As expected by most politicians and sane people, a ridiculous second impeachment failed. Donald Trump has been acquitted. Seven republicans voted for the former president's impeachment and the democrats. The democrats, as expected, were defeated.

The enemy is defeated, the war is won, and all the former president's actions are anathema and will be revised and remade. What to do now? The country is divided into two main irreconcilable camps. Everyone dreams of snatching a piece of a fatter and more prosperous future. It is a once-in-a-lifetime chance to buy a pot of gold with a handful of copper coins. Such a rich bank has never been at stake for world players.

Was that the task of the democrats brings the country to death, get a well-deserved share sufficient for themselves, their grandchildren, and great-grandchildren, and live out a wealthy life in Switzerland or some island paradise? Or maybe there is confusion and dispute in their heads with Napoleonic dreams of universal equality and happiness.

Of course, a large part of the party in the division dream of becoming the masters of this new country, where they will subsequently be masters and have their enslaved people.

The multiple nations that have felt America's weaknesses have their tasks and plan to dispose of assets that have fallen into their hands. It's going to be a feast on the whole world. The truth remains that there are still many American people. Such problems have already been solved, not for the first time. Would it be simpler to collapse the country, the free world leader, as if etched from the inside by some types of insects (beetles, termites), like a mighty 250-year-old tree?

Many enemies who wanted the fall of this country triumphed. China is among the main enemies today.

Instead, the CCP (Chinese Communist Party), the sole ruling party, has established an authoritarian regime since its leader Mao Zedong. In addition to the US on the road to world domination, Donald Trump sought to create a coalition blaming China for the COVID-19 pandemic. Many countries are ready to participate in lawsuits that could balloon to $30 trillion.

WHAT NEXT?

The main question concerns all sane people, not only in the USA. How could it happen, and what awaits the world? How did the Democratic Party pull off such a significant change in the people's minds and practically change the two-party system to the dominant Democratic Party? Judging by the first twenty days of the new government supremacy, it can be confidently called the United States Social-Democratic Party. No one expected such a radical change in the country's domestic and foreign policy. It can be assumed that the forty-sixth president, Joe Biden, went mad and signed multiple documents prepared by America's bribed enemies, his closest aides. The enemy seems to have captured the country and is doing everything to destroy it from within.

Supposedly he behaves like a dictator and does not consult with anyone. His decrees kill jobs and lead to the destruction of an already- dying economy; in that case, Congress should impeach him or remove him from office, freeing up the road for Kamala Harris.

Maybe it was all pre-negotiated, and Joe Biden is the party's new socialist politics executor. Or suddenly, after forty-seven years in the upper echelons of power and nothing special is seen, Joe Biden is a brilliant politician and economist and leads the country to unprecedented success and prosperity? True, this is not consistent with his strange peculiarity of forgetting elementary things and falling into pros-tration at the most inappropriate moment. However, some doubtful people say that Joe Biden, like many of his colleagues, commits all his actions, agreeing to instructions from some intersected sources with a particular influence. Maybe former president Barack Obama is protecting his legacy? Or some sources have provided considerable financial and other services to the right and essential people close to the country's management. Providing services, these sources have particular opportunities to ask politely, or not quite politely, but demand, to provide them with a small service. If this conspiracy theory is correct, then everything becomes simple. The biolog-ical nature of *Homo sapiens* dictates the behavior of the individual.

Food, reproduction, dominance; a person is not a programmed machine with altruistic elements. The desire to create around the oxen sheds pictures of comprehensive happiness, graceful equality, and marvelous celebration of life.

Any person has a certain number of years of stay in this life. If we discard the first twenty years and the last twenty years, people must fulfill their biological purpose in an unreasonably short time.

For someone born rich, beautiful, talented, healthy, and happy, the biological nature and the task are the same as everyone else's. What about those who are unlucky, then what to do? The biological nature and brain suggest a logical solution.

They need to find someone who can help fulfill the purpose, the source that this individual may need. Then it is a matter of technique and ability to adapt to the specified conditions. Opportunities to adapt are observed in some animals and plants. Imitation, the ability to adapt, is the key to success in the chosen field. Possessing such qualities helps *Homo sapiens* break into society's upper classes, even without possessing natural merits.

The most important trait for success is not to be, but to appear. The key to the doors behind which the reward awaits is to show zeal and obedience, which is becoming unavoidable.

Naturally, those born in this life are lucky, and vice versa, those who are unlucky with everything, are the bulk of the world's population.

Even if there are many prerequisites to being wealthy, happy, and prosperous, there is always something that negates a successful pregnancy; careful attention for a woman in labor and the hopes laid down at birth do not succeed. There's always something in the way. It could be the time is incorrect, or the birthplace, relatives, or surroundings, or maybe a person doesn't have the will to achieve something in this life. Sometimes it's all good, but not excellent health from a fate in whole, or a child's appearance may be below expectation.

Appearance is not feet Hollywood's standard hero or heroine. The vast majority are such people—they have their joys and are happy with their fate. Lucky, with an excellent friendly family, lovely children, decent housing, good work, and fun holidays. Who wouldn't want that? It is a life.

Of course, a large group is born with severe dominant character traits. The adventurism of character dictated not paying much attention to the conventional concepts and rules. Morality, correctness, ethics, conscience, and legitimacy in understanding such psycho-types of the human community; these values are only weapons of those who rule others. The goal is to become one of those lucky enough to be one of the strongest in this world, a worthy task. It must be given all the strength and time, stepping over those who stumbled and moving on. Motto: push the one who is falling. It will be an action guide.

In today's society, the upper classes are occupied by the very rich, and they are joined by the famous and people occupying certain places in the political palette of society. Religious leaders do not lag in their influence on many people's minds.

It is a separate caste, and getting into it is not so easy. But to become a political leader, given the modern democratic construction of society, is relatively more straightforward.

Today it is fashionable to be democratic and liberal and close to important people. Express the learned dogma about the good of all segments of the world's population, praise and support all who glorify, and throw thunder and lightning at those who condemn senior fellow party members. Here you are, an elected figure to advance up the hierarchical ladder.

In the United States, two opposing parties have real political force, the Democratic and the Republican Parties.

If you've chosen the Republican Party, you're advocating for freedoms in entrepreneurship, self-regulating free markets, and against government interventions and high taxes. Republicans are in favor of restricting immigration. They support the Second Amendment of the Constitution, the right to buy and bear firearms. They oppose abortion and same-sex marriage. The rights are possible and protect yourself, your family, and your property.

The Democratic Party gravitates toward social

forms of government. It regulates citizens' rights and freedoms—universal and accessible higher education and healthcare. They protect the environment around the planet—and significant taxes on the rich for the fair distribution and maintenance of the poor worldwide.

Democrats oppose gun ownership in favor of undocumented immigrants' rights, the attraction of new migrants, abortion, and same-sex marriage.

Despite opposing views on society's structure, most political parties are united by a single goal: to gain an advantage in the power structures. This rivalry supported the separation of branches of power and the ability to control the power and party, confirming the system of checks and balances recorded in the Constitution of the United States in 1787.

Each party had ideological adherents of the proclaimed doctrine and the goal to achieve these ideals. As is usually the case, people are attached to the movement and more concerned with the simple tasks inherent in the biological nature of *Homo sapiens*, food, reproduction, and dominance. No society, movement, or party can avoid this. The biological essence can be suppressed to force oneself to love others more than your family and to care for the people of another country more than those in one's own country. We can fool others by uttering incendiary speeches and shedding bitter tears on people in

a faraway poor and unhappy country. However, it

is impossible to deceive your biological system. The species of *Homo sapiens* exists today thanks to its survival in the most unfavorable environment.

While in power, members of the Democratic Party, along with the fundamental tasks carried out according to the charter of this party, are subject to the powerful pressure of various corrupt structures, calculating the interests of those who made donations to the funds (funded) the party and the candidate. Corruption and unregulated donations have always existed under the system of electing politicians. Organized crime, foreign states, influential businesses, and transnational organizations make significant contributions, making election campaigns very costly financial processes, the budget of which can be significant.

Famous phrases "we have to pay for everything" and "free cheese only in a mousetrap," is also fair concerning democratically elected representatives of power. From now on, a particular contract binds the giver and the recipient. Failure to fulfill commitments when adopting the "gift" can ruin the relationship. There is also a saying: "Don't spit into the well; you could need a little water to drink" or "May the giver's hand not tremble."

Strive for a high political position; it only makes sense when it's time to "cash in," as Americans say. That is cash out the received dividends. Does this mean that only individuals who seek to meet the biological needs of *Homo sapiens* are naturally sought in politics? Many worthy leaders seek to help society and respect the much-needed rights of all before the law: equality, equal opportunities for all, and the right to freedom, life, and happiness. America was lucky to have such leaders: as George Washington, Abraham Lincoln, Ronald Reagan, and Donald Trump.

YEAR 2021

This year has begun well for the Democratic Party. With a majority in Congress and a democratic president in the White House, the party has decided to rebuild American society. The work was to be grandiose and seemed impossible to many. The party's leaders, led by House Speaker Nancy Pelosi, believed they would do the impossible. The top priority was removing the republican leader, Donald Trump, from the political arena. He was too bright and charismatic around whom resistance could be grouped. Such a confrontation could slow down the process of rebuilding society in the desired liberal-democratic way.

Constitutionally or not, Trump had to be defeated and excluded from political life. He survived the impeachment procedure twice. The main thing for democrats today is not to relax. No, it's not about physically eliminating the main adversary (although, who knows, dreaming is not forbidden to anyone.) The world proletariat leader Josef Stalin quoted a phrase written by the proletarian writer Maxim Gorky: "If the enemy does not give up, it must be destroyed."

Donald Trump is not just an ideological adversary; he is an enemy, severe and dangerous. All is fair in a power war. However, the former president's persona prevents democrats from seeing a bright future that the Democratic Party of the US must build.

Capturing power was a dangerous and challenging task. The Democratic Party could have lost everything if it had been defeated and exposed. During the Clinton and Obama years, the well-established Deep State created the BLM and Antifa strike brigades, a community-trained and organized youth. Luck accompanied the democrats. Everything seemed to be on their side—pandemia, the giants of Silicon Valley, the liberal media, financial tycoons, foreign powers' involvement, and government structures.

But most importantly, mass participation in the election processes of ordinary rank-and-file members of the Democratic Party. While robust structures were orchestrating Donald Trump's ruling administration's downfall, grassroots institutions on the ground were making grandiose fraud by rigging the vote. They were so successful that President Trump, who got an unprecedented seventy-five million votes, was defeated by a new Heracles, Joe Biden, with eighty-two million votes.

Loud statements cannot be; because it simply cannot be, the democrats greeted with anger.

"Let the loser cry, cursing his fate ..." Aria Herman in the opera *The Queen of Spades* by Peter Tchaikovsky.

Having all the trump cards in the new deck of cards, the democrats seriously rebuilt the country under the USA's name (probably temporal). While the party's top focused on fighting the former president, simultaneously declaring all supporters of the former president "domestic terrorists," the new, forty-sixth president, Joe Biden, rolled up his sleeves to sign executive orders, destroying everything that had been created before him.

The country is divided, and a similar situation is explosive. Nobody wants a second Civil War. There will be no winners. Forceful resolution of the problem is more than dangerous. The positions of the sides are diametrically opposite. Simultaneously, a significant destabilizing role is played by multiple minority groups, according to their ideas and objectives.

Dividing the country into a patchwork blanket like Germany at the end of the Second World War will lead to chaos, devastation, and violent opposition. There is simply no real solution to the problem.

Since we mentioned the cards, we should spread

the deck and see "what the day is preparing for us," as is customary for fortune-tellers.

Trying to predict the future is an empty, unproductive occupation, especially on the cards, coffee grounds, the stars, and other little-honored signs.

We can turn to the history of *Homo sapiens* and look for analogies of similar collisions that have taken place in the past with our species.

If we look at the history of the collapse of the ancient Western Roman Empire in the fifth century AD, we will see much research on this subject, combing hundreds of reasons.

Let's highlight the main ones. Political, economic, religious, and cultural. The fall of ancient Rome occurred due to the invasion of external enemies. It is true, but the main reason for the fall was the crisis of Roman society itself.

A large proportion of the population of Rome were barbarians. They were people with different cultures and ideologies. They were attracted by open opportunities to learn to fight. They wanted to fight to take over this rich country.

In Rome, there was a forced slave-owning system. Enslaved people did not want to work for their masters, rebelled, and destroyed all that could be destroyed. Forced higher taxes led to the ruin of agricultural landowners. It affected the economy and trade.

The growth of bureaucracy and civil servants increased corruption and the influence of wealthy people. The devastation of the middle class led to the decline of production, trade, and culture.

The Roman population's moral decay is associated with the popularization of vices, debauchery, attraction to people of the same sex, abandonment of family ties, and reluctance to have children.

Rome was doomed.

The Great French Revolution occurred in 1789 due to the royal authority's inability to solve the state's socioeconomic, political, and financial problems. It was time for changes. The spread of Enlightenment ideas, France's participation in the American Revolution events, crop failure, and famine caused social unrest. The king's power weighed down the clergy, nobility, and bourgeoisie.

The main task was the development of a constitution. The Estates-General Assembly approved the right to vote for all males. Representatives of all estates proclaimed themselves the National Assembly. King Louis XVI was preparing to disperse the national assembly.

"If we have to burn Paris, we will burn Paris."

A cry was shouted: "To arms!" The Guard switched to the people's side. The Paris Commune and the National Guard were born. People broke into the fortress-prison Bastille. King Louis XVI recognized the National Assembly's existence, which became the country's absolute highest authority. The king tried to escape. But he was caught and returned to Paris.

Austrian and Prussian kings announced an armed intervention to restore the monarchy. The National Convention abolished the monarchy and proclaimed France a republic. King Louis XVI was called "enemy and usurper" and sentenced to death. The economic situation continued to deteriorate, and the opponents' armies were advancing, threatening to take over Paris. An era was coming, which would later be called the "era of terror." Suspicious arrests were made, and various committees were "cleansed."

The Revolutionary Tribunal issued a decree on "suspicious" lists. All material and food resources were requisitioned. The newly formed Public Security Committee used the Suspicious Act extensively, sending many of the suspected to the Revolutionary Tribunal.

Terror was politically oriented, pursuing class aliens. Executions were carried out, and mass shootings occurred because the guillotine could not cope. The inter-party struggle began.

After the execution of Danton and his supporters, it was Robespierre' and his supporters' turn. By 1795, the economic crisis had brought inflation to the skies. Widespread hunger and banditry had both become horrific. The united coalition armies of European monarchs were advancing from all sides.

General Bonaparte, who arrived in Paris, was called the savior. An interim government led by Bonaparte was appointed. He subsequently declared himself emperor.

The revolution led to the collapse of the old order, with vast sacrifices to the revolution's development at all stages.

WWI, 1914–1918

Hunger and epidemics due to the war claimed the lives of about twenty million people. The losses are estimated at more than eighteen million lives and about fifty-five million injured. Militaristic Germany opposed France, England, and Russia. In the future, more countries will be drawn into military conflict. The cause of the war was the desire for political and economic domination. In Russia, Vladimir Lenin called for the "transferring of imperialistic war into a civil war." The German General Staff liked the idea, which would withdraw Russia from the coalition, and the Bolsheviks received funding and help to move through the warring European countries to Russia.

In 1917 the monarchy was overthrown in Russia, and power was passed to the Provisional Government. The Bolshevik Party formed armed groups agitating for seizing power among sailors and soldiers. In October, the Bolsheviks overthrew the Provisional Government. Ministers were arrested and sent to the Petropavlovsk fortress prison. A coalition government of the Bolsheviks and leftist Social-Revolutionaries was formed.

Lenin put before the party a "course for radical transformation." A few months later, the Bolsheviks arrested their coalition partners and formed a one-party government. The German-led treaty in Brest in 1918 allowed Germans to liquidate the Western Front.

The decree on the land in 1917 led to confiscation and distribution among the peasants, the landowners, and the church.

Lenin said, "In Paris, the guillotine was working, and we will only deprive of food cards... Let them yell about the arrests. The Tver delegate at the Congress of the Soviets said, 'arrest them all' — that's what I understand; he has an understanding of what the dictatorship of the proletariat is."

Trotsky says that "You can't, they say, sit on bayonets. But you can't do it without bayonets. We need a bayonet there to sit here. All these bourgeois bastards who can now not stand on either side when they learn we're powerful will be with us. The small-bourgeois mass seeks the power it must obey. Those who do not understand this do not understand anything in the world, even less— in the state apparatus."

Mensheviks, right-wing social-revolutionary, SR;

left-wing social-revolutionary, anarchists, and other anti-government organizations were dispersed, and the leaders were arrested.

Decree in the press on October 27, 1917: "All counter-revolutionary newspapers are outlawed."

A "food dictatorship" was announced. Food groups and food armies seized "excess food" from farmers.

A decree on the nationalization of enterprises and the introduction of working control was adopted.

The "military communism" regime was introduced, which led to the complete collapse of industry and rail transport and fleeing to the cities where famine started. Hyperinflation destroyed the monetary emission system.

Labor duty and rationed distribution of goods and services were introduced.

There was widespread resistance to forming armed groups, and the transfer into the Civil War lasted five years.

In this war, everything was confused—reds, whites, invaders, greens, anarchists, socialist revolutionaries, and bandits. The Czechoslovak expeditionary corps, which controlled the Trans-Siberian Railway, rebelled. Troops of German, Austrian, and Romanian interventionists invaded the country. Cossack troops from the Don River, the Ukraine People's Republic, and White-Russia People's Republic (UNR and BPR) rebelled.

Poland, after protracted battles, won independence. The troops of the White Army, under the leadership of the tsar's top commanders, Kolchak, Denikin, Yudenich, Miller, and Wrangel, threatened to seize Moscow. Many regional rebels destabilized the situation, including Kronstadt, Transcaucasia, and Central Asia.

Despite so many well-trained enemies, the Bolsheviks achieved victory. More than fifteen million people were killed in the Civil War. More than two-and-a-half million people left the country.

The worst economic crisis had come. Multiple social groups were on the verge of destruction: military officers, nobility, clergy, Cossacks, and intellectuals.

After the death of the revolution's leader, Vladimir Lenin, in 1924, the power was intercepted by Josef Stalin (Jugashwilli). He was the one who played a crucial role in carrying out repressions. The famous CHK (later KGB) under Felix Dzerzhinsky was renamed the NKVD (People's Commission of Internal Affairs). It was a massive apparatus of intimidation and suppression, carrying out large-scale arrests, torture, shootings, and mass relocation of entire nations; CHK-NKVD had central control of the GULAG (Main Directorate of Correctional Labor Camps.) It prepared fire lists of the "unreliable." The repressed families were also imprisoned in the GULAG camps, and young children were sent to special houses for people without homes. The number of victims of repression is estimated to range in the tens of millions.

The communists used the so-called "doctrine of class struggle,"

approved by Josef Stalin until 1952 (a tyrant's death). The best of the nation, its gene pool, was destroyed.

The people who survived those darkest times included the vile, cunning, able, and loving-to-write denunciations and a silent minority that managed to adapt to everything when the punitive machine destroyed any voice.

It seemed this nightmarish all-present regime would last for centuries. The stagnation of the USSR's socio-economic system quite unexpectedly led to its fall in the late 1980s. The ideology of communism could not stand the test of time and collapse without external interference. Leaving behind the chilling smell of decay after the destruction of its population, the Communist Party of the country saved the mummified effigy of the leader, Vladimir Lenin, in the mausoleum ziggurat in Moscow's Red Square. Despite the collapse of the communist idea in Russia and the seemingly senseless repetition of civil society's model in a communist way, Western politicians still dream of recreating the institutions of a communist utopia. Trying to restore emotions, excitement, and exaltation calls for creating a society where everyone will be equal and happy.

Homo sapiens crave to repeat the unique experience of building a communist society, with an apparent willingness to put under the ax, or the guillotine, those who prevent this dream from being realized.

Another tragic experience creating a totalitarian socialist system was born in a Munich pub on February 24, 1920. Adolf Hitler proclaimed the creation of a new party—the National Socialist German Workers' Party. Nazism—a totalitarian far-right ideology—set the goal of creating a new state for the "Aryan race." According to Hitler, "Socialism is an ancient Aryan German tradition. Our ancestors shared some of the lands."

A program was created to carry out such a historic mission.

The death penalty was introduced against all traitors to the people and the state, the strict authoritarian government of the country. Eliminate any opponents of the regime. One of the essential points is raising youth in the military spirit.

The Nazis tried to come to power by elective means several times but invariably lost. On January 22, 1933, the Reichstag building caught fire. The communists were accused of arson. A "State of Emergency" law was passed. On January 30, Hitler was appointed Reich Chancellor.

Decrees issued: "On the protection of the people and the state," terminating fundamental rights and freedoms. March 13, 1933: Creation of the Ministry of Public Education and Propaganda July 14,

1933: Prohibition or self-dissolution of all political parties except

NSDAP. Law "against the formation of new parties" establishes a one-party state; forming new and continuing political parties became a criminal offense. January 30, 1934: The Empire Reorganization Act eliminated the federal system.

The government had the right to establish new constitutional legislation.

Hitler's socialism in Germany, for twelve years in power, unleashed World War II, where an incredible number of human lives were ruined. The total loss is estimated to be fifty to eighty- million dead.

Southern America has not escaped the influence of the alluring illusions of universal equality. First, the blossoming Cuba, captured by Fidel Castro's rebels, quickly became a third-world country, falling into the USSR's dependence.

Venezuela, the world's most prosperous oil country, was the world's fifth-largest exporter of crude oil. Under the rule of the revolutionary Hugo Chavez from 1998, the promoted socialist nationalization of oil-producing enterprises brought Venezuela to collapse.

SOUTH AFRICA

I n 1652, Dutch sailors transporting spices to Europe arrived in Cape Town. Gradually, the entire territory of the country was conquered by Europeans in battles with African tribes.

Thanks to the discovery of deposits of diamonds and gold, these lands attracted many European and Asian conquerors. The indigenous population of the Bushmen practically disappeared, and some tribes became extinct.

The Afrikaans language combines Dutch (mainstream) with French, German, and Bushman. Almost the entire population in the country speaks Afrikaans.

The British Empire occupied South Africa in 1806. The Dutch who settled in the Cape Town area became farmers and engaged in cattle breeding and agriculture for centuries. The first whites were Portuguese, then primarily Dutch. They were called Afrikaners. Due to a shortage of women, Afrikaners in the Cape Town area engaged in sexual relations with imported enslaved people, forming mixed and transitional races.

The apartheid regime (racial discrimination and segregation) that emerged in 1948 was linked to maintaining white supremacy over large Black populations. It lasted for over forty years.

In May 1994, the first freely elected president of South Africa, Nelson Mandela, was inaugurated. In his inauguration speech, he called for reconciliation and the elimination of racism in South Africa. Nelson Mandela is a Nobel Peace Prize Laureate.

With the transition to democratic rule and active participation of the country's Black population, cases of murder of white farmers increased. Many white people chose to leave.

Dr. Dan Roodt, a professor of literature, described the situation in 2010 as catastrophic, "Today, our people and the rest of South Africa's white population have been the victims of physical and cultural genocide. Over the past fifteen years, more than fifty thousand whites have been killed, and over two hundred thousand of our women have been raped."

THE FUTURE OF THE
USA AND THE WORLD

The events taking place in the United States today will undoubtedly be reflected all over the world. The events that took place in 2020–2021 have shown that the whole world, and the United States, did not expect and did not entirely understand what the country became. As the free world leader, America influenced world politics as a guarantor of democracy and freedom.

Whatever the events that will happen shortly, one thing is clear: America will never be the same. The great dream and the great past have dissipated without a trace. We can only regret the lost dream, draw conclusions, and understand how and why it happened. It must be done if our species, *Homo sapiens*, hope to survive on this planet.

Ideological divisions often end in revolutions and upheavals. Civil wars are fraught with countless casualties and tragedies in people's lives. Irreconcilable differences unambiguously dictate the destruction of opponents. There is too much evil on Earth and a wish to destroy others who do not want to follow other people's rules and desires.

The Founding Fathers created the US on a misguided basis. Slavery cannot be eternal; sooner or later, the enslaved people will rise and destroy the country.

Democracy, as the basis of the political system, is weak and defenseless against the majority's will. It will be a critical moment when most people want changes. Equality is a harmful illusion imposed on the world by Marxists not versed in our species, *Homo sapiens'* biological nature. In any biological species, cubs are born different, with individual capabilities, natural, physical, and data, and develop under different circumstances. *Homo sapiens* are no exception. Our species, passing the long and bloody path of biological survival in nature, has found the most favorable survival system: to stick together in a flock.

People aren't born the same. They have learned to think and interact with each other. The history of our species' civilization for five millennia of its existence, up to the twenty-first century, displays slavery, the destruction of humankind with wild cruelty, forced obedience, the use of false theories and lies, beautiful fairy tales, and slogans. The advent of the twenty-first century changed nothing about it, but the fairy tales and slogans have become more refined.

The essence has not changed. Herd instinct and fear of an unknown future make people believe in the ideas preached by false prophets. Religion gave hope for protection and a fair trial in the afterlife.

The false prophets of Karl Marx's ideology promise equality for all, not only before the law but in the foreseeable future, but if, of course, the evil greedy capitalist bloodsuckers will not interfere with the society of equal opportunities.

If we try again to make a society of equal opportunities, where everyone is happy, cheerful, and healthy, isn't it just beautiful?

American democrats led people to deception, forgery, and crime, turning the 2020 election into a farce and a mockery of justice. They don't think so.

> Even if there were some inaccuracies, the great goal
> of creating a society of equal opportunity justifies any
> action leading to the creation of the common good.

They don't think so; they say so. The goal is straightforward, power.

The *Homo sapiens* species cannot change its biological nature. Power is the road to food sources, the successful continuation of our family, and the purpose is fulfillment—predominance.

Two parties constantly fight for control over the USA, republicans and democrats;—each party has a certain amount of control over the other to prevent violations of the Constitution. It was laid out by the Founding Fathers to prevent the possibility of tyranny. But if one party gains total control over all branches of government, what happens, then? Here are the possibilities.

To send to other countries financial help all around the globe. It is easy to imagine what gratitude awaits those who get this terrific help. Any country needs the latest military equipment to win the war. It's all money, and what a great deal of money.

It is possible to fight climate warming; however, it has been cold. Money can and should be printed. However, the country's debt is approaching a sky-high $30 trillion, which must be paid sooner or later. But not today. The pandemic happened so well, thanks to the Chinese Communist Party. People should not relax, gather in groups, rally, or talk nonsense. The quarantine is a beautiful remedy for chatter.

Suppose someone thinks that in the 2022 midterm elections or the 2024 presidential election, mistakes made in 2020 can be corrected, then they are wrong. The Democratic Party did not put existence on the line in the 2020 elections to allow that power to be taken away from them.

If the Democrats lose, they will be blamed for everything they have done. Seizure of power. Millions of falsifications and vote-rigging in the counting of votes. The shame and intimidation of elite politicians, law enforcement officers, courts up to the country's Supreme Court, the military, and lawyers. Anyone who sided with Trump.

The media, loyal to democratic candidates, did accuse Trump supporters of declaring them "domestic terrorism." It was a coup d'état. Suppose the democrats lose momentum and allow the Republican Party to take power away. In that case, there is a clear and unconditional danger of falling under the pressure of criminal procedure legislation.

Democrats are not fools. They would lose everything. They risk losing their jobs and fortunes and going to jail as a result.

The de facto Democratic Party managed to pull off such a daring power-grabbing operation in 2020 right under the noses of the unsuspecting Republican Party. That means they have talented strategists who can plan a nationwide operation with international assistance. They will fight for power, using all the possibilities, checking in the history books how those who successfully stood up in the power struggle acted under similar circumstances.

The main task is to keep power, preferably forever, at all costs. The stakes in the game are very high. The forty-sixth president, Joe Biden, is ready and willing to stand like a rock. It's not only about his beloved son, Hunter Biden, and the president himself. Joe Biden is president, and no one dared to cause him evil or take

away what he earned; for this, he went to the presidency. Although he understood that he had almost no
chance to handle this position correctly, he was not
getting any younger.

*He has already earned everything he needs, but there is never
too much money. He probably would rather play with the dog,
sleep until noon, and kiss his grandchildren. But the party said:
You must! We will do everything. Sit, and do not stand out too
much; otherwise, God forbid, you will get sick at your age. Do
what we say, and you will be happy. We're going to do all of it.*

Joe Biden may want to retire, but those who bet on
him want to get their dividends.

The Biden family's ties to Russia and China are
under investigation. Fox News reported that US senators involved in the investigation into Hunter Biden's
business contacts have new data confirming the US
president-elect's family's ties to Russia and China.
Simultaneously, republican congressman Ralph
Norman complained that democrats do not want to
investigate the American channel's air.

Congressman Ralph Norman: "Let's examine this
just-published report excerpt. Grassley and Johnson
state, 'These new data confirm not only the existence
of ties between the Biden family and the communist
Chinese government, but also between Hunter
Biden's business partners and the Russian government.
But also, information from the committee's September
23, 2020 report raised concerns on the counterintelligence line and in terms of possible extortions.'"

This information is not only essential but should also be alarming. If a member of Joe Biden's family did receive money from a company associated with the Chinese government, for that money would have to be accounted for. Among the government representatives from the democratic government, other names are known for their ties with China. Among them is Representative Eric Swalwell, who participated in the democratic primaries as a candidate for the United States president. He was the manager and co-actor in President Trump's impeachment. When he sat on the House Intelligence Committee, he was directly connected with the Chinese communist spy Christine Fang.

Senator Dianne Feinstein of California, who served as the senior democrat on the Senate Judiciary Committee, and is the former mayor of San Francisco, was reprimanded for employing her driver for twenty years as a Chinese citizen.

Senate Republican majority leader Mitch McConnell accused Trump of provoking a crowd on January 6, 2021, during an intrusion into the Capitol Building.

Elaine Chao, the second wife of Mitch McConnell, was Secretary of Transportation. Her family's shipping company, The Foremost Group, has close ties to the Chinese elite.

Tom Brenner, the New York Times:

"The Chinese trail is everywhere in colleges, economics, politics, in investment projects. The trade volume between China and the United States reached $385.3 billion in 2010."

At the end of 2011, trade amounted to $456.8 billion, with a surplus of $273 billion in favor of China. The US-China trade war began in 2018. The United States and China are fighting two different strategies for world leadership.

In August 2020, US President Donald Trump said that he did not rule out a complete cessation of economic cooperation with China under certain conditions.

In an interview on Fox News, Trump responded to a question host about whether the US economy can allow separation from the Chinese. According to the American leader, the American economy suffered huge losses because of Beijing.

In a statement, William Evanina, director of the US National Counterintelligence and Security Center, said, "China does not support Trump's re-election, which Beijing considers 'unpredictable.' In the run-up to the November elections, China was trying to "form a political environment in the United States, to put pressure on politicians whose position, in his opinion, contradicts the interests of China."

"Of course they want Biden. I took billions of dollars from China and gave them to our farmers and the US Treasury. China will own the US if Biden and Hunter [Joe Biden's son] join it," Trump wrote.

A Chinese scholar living in the United States

wrote: "The Communist Party of China (CPC) is probably the most ideologically intoxicated, dogmatic Political Party of the Leninist ideology in the history of mankind."

"The CPC wants to replace the US-controlled international order with its authoritarian governance model, and their internal definition of the United States as a major adversary has never changed."

China does not want to exacerbate confrontation with the United States. However, there are areas in which there will be no compromise—first of all, ideology, power of the CPC, most issues of domestic policy, the system of governance of the state, issues of national security and territorial integrity, and more.

In the US, lobbying is legal and strictly regulated by law. The Secretary of the Senate or the Clerk of the House of Representatives has informed the customers of lobbying services, lobbying decisions, and the amounts received by lobbyists. There is a link between donations to individual lawmakers' electoral funds and legislative decisions that lobbyists and sponsors were interested in. The Chinese lobby focuses on the solid economic dependence of entire economic sectors of the PRC market.

Wikipedia: The establishment is the foundation - those in power, ruling circles, political elite.

People with high social and political positions are

the most important in the existing social system. They're forming public opinion and social foundations through which these people maintain the existing social courses. Like Biden's son, the son of Nancy Pelosi, after the overthrow of the legal regime of Yanukovych, it turned out that he was engaged in business in Ukraine. Nancy Pelosi went to Ukraine in 2015 to discuss "energy security," NRGLab was interested in gas production in Ukraine before the coup. In 2017, Paul Pelosi, as a representative of Viscoil and NRGLab, went to Ukraine, ostensibly to discuss cooperation in the "sphere of football."

A 2013 YouTube commercial shows Nancy Pelosi and her son discussing energy-saving technology benefits.

Pop-up details of how the American establishment (primarily the leadership of Democrats—Clinton, Biden, Pelosi) was embroiled in Ukrainian corruption at the highest level.

PRESIDENT JOE BIDEN

In the first month of his presidency, Joe Biden signed over fifty executive orders overturning the Trump administration's decisions. Such a decisive turn in domestic and foreign policy has caused concern and worry, especially in those states where coal, oil, and gas are mined.

Apparent resistance in some states is causing Biden's intention to eliminate the Second Amendment to the Constitution. That is the right to purchase and carry firearms. Even more strongly resisted are the decrees in migration policy changes—amnesty for illegal immigrants (according to various estimates from eleven to twenty-five million) and obtaining citizenship. Biden had a problem canceling the wall's construction on the border with Mexico (a third of the wall has been built).

A family reunion of illegal immigrants; thousands

of illegal immigrant families were separated by deportation from the USA to commit different crimes. President Joe Biden proposed the priority of reunification for such families.

All of this legislation aims to increase the potential electoral base for the Democratic Party. However, it contributes to increased crime and drug smuggling into the US, many republicans said.

All of it led to the following.

Repealing the rule for migrants about separation from children when illegally crossing the border.

Cancellation of deportation for 100 days for convicted illegal migrants.

The lifting of the travel ban, set by Trump, on people from several Muslim countries.

Introduction of relief for those who want to get asylum in the US.

"This biased proposal rewards those who have broken the law, floods the labor market at a time when millions of Americans are unemployed, unable to secure the border, and encourages further illegal immigration," lawmaker Jim Jordan said.

Results In New
Reality

Irreconcilable differences in the vision of American society's future can cause the country to disintegrate into two or more parts. There are many reasons for such a sad ending. Whether such disengagement could be peaceful enough or without shedding blood is up to those ready for extreme measures or express readiness for a peaceful resolution through negotiations.

Perhaps today's generation has reached a critical mass after centuries of society's established structure of capitalism. Some people got incredibly rich, but some were very poor. Society no longer wants to put up with the existing situation. Or it could be that the propaganda of social society with equality and social benefits, the same for all, found grateful followers. People say no to a society of rich and poor.

Freedom, equality, and brotherhood! It seems it was said before. "The new is a well-forgotten old one."

Main contradictions in American society:

Classes: Ideological, Racial, National, Religious, Gender, Equality, Cultural.

The difference between the super-rich and the frankly poor has reached its climax. The traditional billionaires of the Forbes magazine list have been added to giants with social networks and new technologies. Jeff Bezos, founder and CEO of Amazon, 2021, the wealthiest man, owns a net capital of $193.4 billion. By comparison, the poverty rate in the US is skyrocketing. The COVID-19 pandemic has dramatically increased the vulnerable population as tens of millions of Americans have lost their businesses, jobs, homes, and health insurance. The city streets are filled with homeless people and beggars for various reasons. Lack of confidence in the future, fear for the family, and an unknown future push people to extreme measures.

Ideology: Such contradictions are connected with the lack of a clear understanding of what system of governance of society meets the average American's requirements. Having some knowledge about socialistic state systems, it becomes evident that something is not working. Such regimes hold on to the dictatorship, infringing fundamental rights and freedoms, lowering the standard of living, and suppressing the individual.

The American way of life, the American dream of

owning a home, a successful job or a business, a happy family, freedom of speech, and the inalienable rights of a free citizen are ideal for most Americans. Democrats offer their vision for a country where everyone is equal and happy.

Those who voted for the Democratic Party are willing to sacrifice certain human rights for a tolerable existence.

RACIAL

Slavery as a factor of American society has been laid down in the country's foundation. This disparity between Black and white people cannot be settled by simple handouts in reparations and preferential rights when entering higher education, employment, or higher legal positions. Democrats are trying to solve this problem by paying enormous reparations for the years of slavery. But the split in society is too great. Centuries of suffering, trampling on pride, lack of conditions for society's development, and racial genocide are impossible to forget. Reparations will not solve this problem. Today, there is simply no solution to this problem.

RELIGIOUS

Although some religious doctrines have lost their ferocity and call on the flock to resolve consent, the religious divisions that have existed since the totem primitive society are too great.

The last question was especially worried about by the Founding Fathers of the American state. The US Constitution defines religion as a private matter for every citizen and insists on a clear separation of church and religious state. The First Amendment to the US Constitution prohibits Congress from passing laws establishing any religion or prohibiting its free practice.

Violent religious movements are a trap that convinces the followers of the truth of the learned postulates. Radical Islam has many religious movements. The Muslim population in the United States 2021 will be about four million. Radical Islam is popular among African Americans, which continues the famous Nation of Islam activities.

Gender equality

Today's America promotes other values, putting the plurality of the sexes first. The biological genders of males and females are no longer traditional, well-established representations in today's social culture. Accordingly, the grammar must change, emphasizing the gender chosen by the individual. Adapting to the new culture, the family should not prevent the child from choosing his gender, the child's identification in society, and support the child in his decision. The species of *Homo sapiens* has already experienced a similar phenomenon of social culture. The ancient Roman Empire was distinguished by an extreme degree of perversion; true, this did not save her from falling. Scientists who studied ape behavior during puberty observed homosexuals (or, as we should express in new, modern behavior, people attracted to some members of the same gender). *Homo sapiens* have inherited their ancestors' gay preferences, which are the norm today.

CULTURAL

Multiculturalism is equivalent to a clash of civilizations. Various socialities created different races and peoples' cultures, traditions, everyday conditions of nature, customs, religions, levels of knowledge, philosophy, art, music, and literature. The system of values in the culture of one civilization can cause rejection in another. Every culture defends its absolute truths. Each religion sees itself as the last resort's truth with all the logical consequences that follow and reasonably practical consequences in the confessional states.

All of the above contradictions will contribute to the disintegration of the country. The critical mass of the population, demanding drastic change, has reached a level where such changes are inevitable. It remains to be hoped that such disruption will be achieved without bloody upheavals.

Such an example of disintegration in the recent history of our species, *Homo sapiens*, occurred in 1991 in the USSR. With the Union of Soviet Socialist Republics, the treaty signed by representatives of the three republics, Russia, Ukraine, and Belorussia, liquidated the former union and created the (CIS) Commonwealth of Independent States.

The reasons for this disintegration were ideological, economic, and national. Mass movements for national independence rocked the "socialist power ship," and disintegration became inevitable.

The referendum held in the country supported the creation of the CIS. It happened without bloodshed, peacefully. If the country's disintegration is inevitable, we must hope for the warring parties' prudence and the peaceful resolution of emerging conflicts.

In Texas, a House of Representatives member, Republican Kyle Biedermann, proposed a referendum on secession from the United States. He believes that the federal government is out of control and no longer represents the value of Texans.

The ruling elite of the Democratic Party, following the instincts of *Homo sapiens* and realistically assessing the danger threatened from the unpredictable and uncontrollable President Donald Trump, skillfully and resolutely went on the offensive. The upcoming 2020 presidential election predicted a victory for "sitting" President Donald Trump, which meant another four years of him in the White House.

All previous attempts with allegations of ties to Russia or pressure on the president of Ukraine fell apart in the Senate, where Republicans had a majority. Trump's threat was evident and present danger. Having shaken off the attacking democrats from himself, like a pack of dogs being thrown away by an angry bear, he could go on the offensive, and it was impossible to allow such a thing.

Trump has repeatedly stated that he intends to disperse the "Washington swamp." There, the heads of more significant and very influential people could fly.

Someone could end up in prison and lose a collected fortune; many could lose personal connections, a brilliant career, or an expensive income while building wealthy and essential positions for their own children. In short, it could have been a disaster. Trump was doomed. Palace coups, intrigues, and the power struggle accompany the entire history of Homo sapiens. Dominance has never been canceled. The democrats decided on a coup d'état. It could be dangerous. They could be accused of mutiny and the violent overthrow of the legally elected government. They could lose everything or even end up in the dock. True, inaction meant another four years of President Trump's rule, threatening the possible loss of everything and for everyone. Some influential persons had obligations (perhaps financial, dependence on obligations) in specific circles. The one who pays calls the tune. Maybe some skeletons in the closet can't be brushed off. Addiction is a demanding fate. One of the Roman senators Cato Senior, finishing his speech on any topic, always said, "And Carthage must be destroyed." As well, democrats, talking about Trump, always mentioned his bad qualities, actions, and character traits as inappropriate for the presidency. Developing a victorious path to remove Donald Trump from the presidency in four years was necessary.

The conspirators developed a brilliant strategy, with interested foreign countries' participation, attracted to their side strike groups of rebels (Antifa, BLM).

They placed the right people in all critical areas of power, up to the Supreme Court. Those who could not be bribed were intimidated by the militants.

Liberal media and social networks, forgetting about all amendments in the Constitution, issued false propaganda and blocked all who tried to prove otherwise. "Necessary" voting machines were purchased, with programs that allowed them to "correct" undesirable results.

So, by the way, came the COVID-19 pandemic, making it possible to legally lock the population at home and ensuring voting would be conducted by mail.

Nevertheless, there were many troubling moments when an almost clear victory could have been lost. With predictable luck in courts, the right people and the authorities in the right states, though republicans,

RESULTS IN NEW REALITY

knew what to do. One troubling moment is when the full-state Congress approves the electorate's votes and the presidential nomination. Vice-president-presiding Mike Pence could overturn the fragile structure and nullify many people's efforts and considerable money. This task was solved.

Another brilliant plan allowed the United States presidency to approve the necessary candidacy and permanently eliminate an opponent such as Donald Trump from the political arena. Something similar to storming the Bastille in France or the Winter Palace in Russia. It will be more accessible to approve the right president and accuse Donald Trump as the rebellion's initiator, with the threat of the lives of those in power. The necessary candidacy is approved, and Trump faces another impeachment with the threat of a ban on ever holding elected office. As Americans say: kill two birds with one stone.

Stormtroopers Antifa easily coped with the trifling assault. On the contrary, the police guarding the people's representatives did not resist but invited people to enter. With good reason and confidence in his rightness, Vice President Mike Pence approved the victory of the democratic president.

Impeachment number two did not fly because, despite the betrayal of several republicans, the Senate acquitted President Trump, for the prosecution required 67 percent of the vote. However, it was a victory. Both houses of Congress and the White House were in the hands of the democrats. The democrats won not only the battle but the entire "crusade."

What was left to fulfill the next, no less necessary task was to leave the rule of power for the foreseeable future, preferably forever.

As the forty-sixth president of the United States shows poorly hidden signs of memory loss, it is not surprising. The first month of Joe Biden's presidency left no doubt about the strategy.

As if he was selected to perform a particular task, his rather strange team brings several decrees daily to the head of state, which he signs with evident pleasure, though he sometimes asks: What do I sign?

It's become noticeable that democrats were concerned and decided to change the control system on the so-called nuclear "red button."

During his first month in office, President Joe Biden *knocked over* almost all of the Trump administration's *"accomplishments."* It's more like *"the entourage is playing the king."*

Perhaps Vice President Kamala Harris is acting in the shadow of the *"screen president."*

Destructive decrees, one after another, eliminated jobs in a balanced economy. It may be a solution to the country's power problem. A bet on a "Green New Deal" pushed by a former Bronx barmaid and now congresswoman AOC, the ideological leader of the so-called Squad of Four in the House of Representatives, pushed the country back.

Changes in immigration laws are aimed at a significant increase in the number of migrants entering the country. Return to all the agreements which Trump's administration pulled out.

Respect for the legal rights of racial, religious, people with non-traditional orientation, and the rights of LGBT communities.

Preparations for payments as reparations for the families of victims during slavery times were moving ahead.

The allocation of $1.9 trillion to stimulate the pandemic hit the US economy, in which much of the package aims went to help other countries.

Only a fraction of President Joe Biden's executive orders were signed in the first month of the new president's term. Almost all of the forty-sixth president's decrees aim to destroy the country's economy and send financial aid to other countries.

Naturally, there are many questions. Does the government understand what it is doing? What is the purpose of all this destructive management? Who benefits from a weak, divided America?

All those who want to weaken the influence of the United States? All who want to change the dollar monetary system of the world? Is introducing all electronic currency, including Bitcoin types, just a matter of time?

It would seem silly to ruin the economy and destroy the dollar monetary system. It is equivalent to sawing the branch on which we are sitting. However, for many, especially those playing on short (Soros, China, bankers, financial tycoons), such a collapse of the giant US economy is a gift from a well-prepared operation. To buy collapsed assets for next to nothing, wait for the rise, sell, and earn fabulous profits.

In any case, democrats must destroy the country to keep power in perspective.

That is from a scary nightmare. Democrats will not allow this; they won't give up power just like that.

They cannot afford to lose power in the next elections. It could be a disaster for anyone involved in a coup: courts, prisons, losses of everything.

They took a chance and won. As one foolish man used to say, "I'll bet 100 bucks against a bagel hole; you don't think it will happen."

Democrats know they will stay in power only by destroying the country. It will be possible to easily change the country's constitution, securing one party's rule forever. Instantly impoverished, the hungry population will seek protection and salvation in power.

If living in one big country is pretty dangerous, it could be possible to agree, as was done in Russia, and divide into separate unions. There was already a precedent. North and South. The Confederate States vs. the United States.

Make your bets, ladies and gentlemen!

Epilogue

Democrats and those who have worked out and developed plans of power grab naturally consider all the difficulties and possible options to counter such plans. It will be a massive country with almost 333 million people by 2020, with fifty federal and independent states. With many firearms on hand, owned by people accustomed to freedom and pride for their country, it would be strange to assume that they will voluntarily lay down their arms, put their hands behind their backs, and go voluntarily into a new and dark tomorrow. It is the first, but not the last, problem.

The second is a no less complex problem, many minorities, each requiring building a new society according to their preferences. They are promised a lot, but these minorities are poorly managed, noisy, and always ready to exacerbate the situation. Such separatism requires an extraordinary approach.

Finally, just a democratic population of the country supporting the ideas of democracy or even socialism. So far, so good; they shout hooray and toss their hats up. Nobody knows how they will behave when they "smell something bad."

Dividing into two or even three independent entities is possible. The main thing is to avoid bloodshed. Allow each sovereign state to implement its social policy, economy, and the protection of its borders. If it happened in Russia, it could be possible in America.

Such a country's partition threatens substantial financial losses, the lost status of great power, and many mangled destinies.

But this is the best fate has to offer this country.

I have read the above countless times and concluded that everything is outdated. Today's life is fast current, and events become obsolete the next day. Today, everything that was important and required attention and reflection seems naive and unnecessary. Humanity in its history has gone through many radical changes in its destiny. There were important and necessary stages of our species' development, but changes often led to wars and the destruction of entire populations and continents. One era ended, and another came.

Can the year 2020 be considered a landmark year in our species? We will see.

In the past, an era of absolute monarchism did give way to a bourgeois parliamentary system.

In inventing the theory of "surplus value," Karl Marx pointed the way to a socialist revolution and a radical transformation of the social order.

Post-war Europe chose a political system, a democratic parliamentary form of government. Our era has brought many bloody upheavals—two world wars with unthinkable human casualties.

Some states preferred a constitutional monarchy.

Russia has been transformed into a socialist state.

The United States, since its inception, has been a federal presidential republic whose constitution enshrined the principle of separation of powers. Legislative, executive, and judicial branches were acting under the Constitution independently.

The Constitution guaranteed fundamental political rights: freedom of speech, freedom of assembly, religion, and freedom of the press. The preamble of the Constitution recognized the people as the source of power. Life dictated its terms, and twenty-seven constitutional amendments were adopted. Thus, all population segments, including all minorities, have the same rights. The people choose their representatives, relying on their opinions on election promises and views on their social structure.

The Republican Party founded more than a quarter of a century later, has long been the country's ruling party, thanks to Abraham Lincoln in the Civil War. Personal freedom and free enterprise made this country the leader of the free world.

The presidencies of the democratic candidates, Clinton (1992—2000) and Barack Obama (2008—2016), had a significant impact on the country, which suddenly began to change dramatically in the United States and the entire planet.

Global crises developed out of control and changed everything.

In-country changes happened in ethnic, racial, religious, gender, social, cultural, and intellectual structures.

In 2020, most of the US population voted for the democratic nominee.

There was a bloodless revolution that would radically change the whole world.

A new era is coming.

GRATITUDE

For work on this book, I used materials published in the media, public lectures, debates of candidates participating in the US election campaign, politicians' speeches, and scientists. Also, various sources of information are widely available in the public domain.

The first chapter of this part of the book focuses on the Russian scientist and doctor of biological sciences, professor Savelev Sergey Vyacheslavovich's research and writings. All rights to these printed works belong to the publishing house VEDI. Professor Sergey Savelev is a paleo-neurologist evolutionist and head of the Russian Academy of Sciences human nervous system morphology laboratory. The author of numerous books, lectures, and speeches on radio and television, a scientist with comprehensive knowledge, devoted his life to studying the human brain. His modern ideas regarding the human brain, implacable position of defending his opinion, and somewhat bold and innovative thoughts about today's society brought him many fans, opponents, and critics. It explains the causes that led to the loss of a modern man's brain volume of an average of 50 to 280 cubic centimeters.

Courtesy of VEDI publishing
The End of *Homo Sapiens* Vol III